Dermatological Diseases
of the Nose and Ears

Can Baykal
K. Didem Yazganoğlu

Dermatological Diseases of the Nose and Ears

An Illustrated Guide

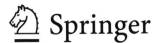

Prof. Dr. Can Baykal
Dr. K. Didem Yazganoğlu
Istanbul University
Istanbul Medical Faculty
Department of Dermatology
Millet Cad CAPA
34390 Istanbul
Turkey
baykalc@istanbul.edu.tr
karadidem@yahoo.com

ISBN: 978-3-642-01558-8   e-ISBN: 978-3-642-01559-5

DOI: 10.1007/978-3-642-01559-5

Springer Heidelberg Dordrecht London New York

Library of Congress Control Number: 2009934483

© Springer-Verlag Berlin Heidelberg 2010

This work is subject to copyright. All rights are reserved, whether the whole or part of the material is concerned, specifically the rights of translation, reprinting, reuse of illustrations, recitation, broadcasting, reproduction on microfilm or in any other way, and storage in data banks. Duplication of this publication or parts thereof is permitted only under the provisions of the German Copyright Law of September 9, 1965, in its current version, and permission for use must always be obtained from Springer. Violations are liable to prosecution under the German Copyright Law.

The use of general descriptive names, registered names, trademarks, etc. in this publication does not imply, even in the absence of a specific statement, that such names are exempt from the relevant protective laws and regulations and therefore free for general use.

Product liability: The publishers cannot guarantee the accuracy of any information about dosage and application contained in this book. In every individual case the user must check such information by consulting the relevant literature.

Cover design: Frido Steinen-Broo, eStudio Calamar, Figueres/Berlin

Printed on acid-free paper

Springer is part of Springer Science+Business Media (www.springer.com)

Preface

Books concerning regional approaches to dermatological diseases always create great enthusiasm among physicians, and can be very useful resources for dermatologists. Lesions on the nose and ears are commonly observed in daily clinical practice. Thanks to their prominent location, they are noticed earlier by the patients; therefore, patients very frequently seek earlier medical attention. Diseases with different pathogenesis may occur in these regions and they sometimes require a multidisciplinary approach. Based upon these facts, I thought that a book specific to dermatological diseases of the nose and ears would be useful in the daily practice of different specialists. The story of this book started approximately 10 years ago, with my special interest in patients with pemphigus vulgaris localized to the nose. I then started to gather clinical material about the dermatological diseases of the nose. As some diseases of the external ear also have common features with the diseases of the nose, I also collected material about the dermatological diseases of the ear. In the end I decided to share my experience with my colleagues through a book. Thereafter, I collaborated with Dr. K. Didem Yazganoğlu from my department. After positive review of the first version of the book in Turkish, we decided to prepare an international edition. The interest of Springer-Verlag made this possible.

This book provides summarized information about almost all dermatological diseases that affect the nose and the ears. The text is focused on clinical features and some diagnostic clues about these diseases. The book is divided into two sections: diseases of the nose and diseases of the ears. It includes 19 chapters. The name of each chapter indicates the most common dermatological elementary lesions which will be discussed. Therefore, diseases presenting with a predominant type of elementary lesion are discussed in the related chapter. As a result, almost 600 different diseases of the skin are presented in this book. However, the information given about the diseases affecting both regions are not repeated in each section. Twenty two books and internet sources (pubmed) were accessed to optimize the topics and to select all the dermatological diseases affecting the nose and ears for this book.

Initially, physicians may observe or be concerned about a simple nose or ear lesion. After identifying the specific elementary lesion, they can more easily uncover the diagnosis of local or disseminated disease with the guidance of this book. Four hundred and twenty-eight original photographs have been used to assist the clinician for a quick diagnosis. We have included high quality images from our own files, most of them photographed by us and 28 photographs were obtained from our colleagues in other departments. This book's primary target audience are both beginners and the experts of the two disciplines – dermatology and ear-nose and throat diseases. Plastic surgeons or general practitioners who treat cutaneous diseases may also have a particular interest in this book. We hope that this book will help clinicians in diagnosing challenging cases.

Can Baykal

Acknowledgements

We thank our colleagues in the Dermatology Department and the Dermatopathology Unit of the Pathology Department in Istanbul Medical School for their contribution to the diagnosis of the challenging cases included in this book.

Contents

The Importance of the Nose from a Dermatological Point of View
The Anatomy of the Nose 1

    1 Macular Lesions 3
    2 Vesiculobullous and Pustular Lesions. 11
    3 Eczematous and Squamous Lesions 17
    4 Hyperkeratotic Lesions 23
    5 Papular Lesions 27
    6 Nodular Lesions 37
    7 Granulomatous Lesions 53
    8 Deformities 59
    9 Ulcerative Lesions 69

The Importance of the Ear from a Dermatological Point of View
The Anatomy of the Ear 75

    10 Macular Lesions 77
    11 Vesiculobullous and Pustular Lesions. 85
    12 Eczematous and Squamous Lesions 91
    13 Hyperkeratotic Lesions 99
    14 Papular Lesions 103
    15 Nodular Lesions 111
    16 Granulomatous Lesions 131
    17 Deformities 135
    18 Ulcerative Lesions 143
    19 Hypertrichosis 147

References 149

Index 151

Physicians who have Contributed Images to the Book

Dr. Oya Gürbüz (Marmara University Medical School), Fig. 1.3

Dr. Pamir Erdinçler (Cerrahpaşa Medical School), Fig. 6.1

Dr. Ayşe Kavak (Düzce University Medical School), Figs. 6.25, 15.11, 15.41

Dr. Mustafa Sütlaş (Istanbul Leprosy Hospital), Figs. 7.4, 16.6, 16.7, 16.8

Dr. Ertan Yılmaz (Akdeniz University Medical School), Fig. 7.9

Dr. Bilal Doğan (GATA Haydarpaşa Hospital), Fig. 8.23, 9.15

Dr. Soner Uzun (Çukurova University Medical School), Figs. 9.2, 16.9, 18.7, 18.8

Dr. Erkan Alpsoy (Akdeniz University Medical School), Fig. 9.8

Dr. Dilek Bayramgürler (Kocaeli University Medical School), Fig. 13.7

Dr. Deniz Seçkin (Başkent University Medical School), Fig. 14.4

Dr. Orhan Aral (Istanbul Medical School), Figs. 14.6, 14.7

Dr. Tülin Mansur (Haydarpaşa Numune Hospital), Figs. 14.13, 14.14, 15.21

Dr. Ümmühan Kaya (Dermatologist in private practice), Fig. 15.24

Dr. Ayşen Karaduman (Hacettepe University Medical School), Fig. 15.32

Dr. Tülin Ergun (Marmara University Medical School), Fig. 17.19

Dr. Özlem Dicle (Akdeniz University Medical School), Fig. 19.4

Images listed below were used in the book entitled "Dermatoloji atlası (Atlas of Dermatology)," of C. Baykal (2004): 1.3, 1.10, 1.18, 2.7, 3.7, 3.11, 4.5, 5.4, 5.5, 5.6, 5.17, 6.3, 6.6, 6.13, 6.23, 6.35, 6.37, 6.39, 6.45, 6.47, 6.49, 7.1, 7.11, 7.14, 8.11, 8.12, 8.21, 8.24, 8.25, 9.6, 9.10, 10.21, 11.6, 11.13, 12.7, 12.22, 13.3, 13.9, 13.13, 14.3, 14.8, 14.12, 14.15, 14.20, 15.15, 15.20, 15.25, 15.53, 15.58, 15.60, 15.65, 16.3, 17.9.

Images listed below were used in the book entitled "Dermatoloji'de algoritmik tanı (Algoritmic diagnosis in Dermatology)", of VL. Aksungur, E. Alpsoy, C. Baykal, S. Uzun (2007): 2.2, 6.27, 6.44, 8.1, 9.8, 9.11, 13.4, 15.13, 19.6.

Figure 7.9 was used in the manuscript of Akman A et al.: "Cutaneous rhinosporidiosis presents with recurrent nasal philtrum mass in Southern Turkey," Int J Dermatol 2008 Jul;47(7):700-3.

NOSE

The Importance from a Dermatological Point of View

Part of the face

An acral region

A periorificial region

Part of the midline

A region densely exposed to ultraviolet light

An intertriginous surface

A region innerved by trigeminal nerve

A seborrheic region

A cartilaginous region

A region showing congenital deformity in genodermatoses

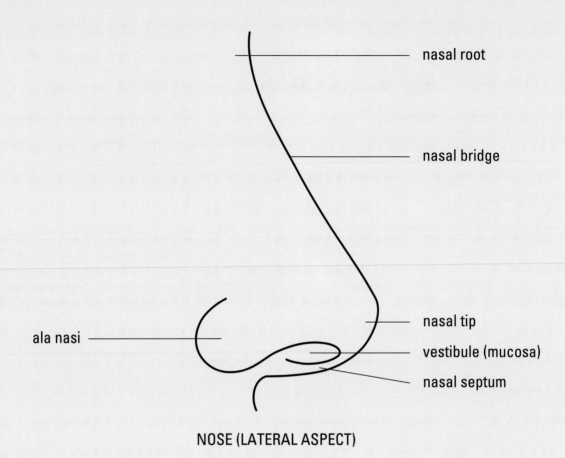

NOSE (LATERAL ASPECT)

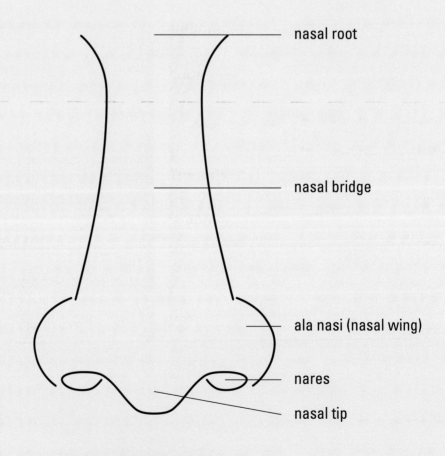

NOSE (ANTERIOR ASPECT)

1 ■ Macular Lesions

Macules are flat lesions that show discolouration. The prominent facial position of the nose allows the nasal macular lesions easily be noticed. Hyperpigmented macules on the nose may have different causes. Fixed drug eruption is mostly seen around the mouth and eyelids, however it can also occur as sharply-defined, grey-brown coloured, round or oval macules on the nose. There is often a previous history of inflammatory nummular erythema at the same site. While cotrimoxazole and naproxen are the most common causative agents in fixed drug eruption, a large spectrum of medications can induce these lesions. Drug-induced hyperpigmentation, caused by drugs like amiadarone, quinidine and antimalarials, can affect the nose together with the cheeks and forehead. Such pigmentation is often bluish grey in colour (Fig. 1.1). Clofazimine, which is used for the treatment of leprosy, can induce a diffuse pigmentation that may be prominent on the nose. Hyperpigmentation on the nose together with other sun-exposed sites of the face can occur after PUVA therapy (Fig. 1.2). Facial hyperpigmentation of melasma, which is typically located on the forehead, cheeks, chin and around the lips, can also involve the nose. This common cosmetic problem is primarily seen in women and may occur during pregnancy. Typical light-brown patches have irregular borders.

Skin lesions of ochronosis (alkaptonuria) which result from the deposition of homogentisic acid are most likely to occur prominently in middle age. The persistent irregular pigmentation is greyish or bluish black in colour, located mostly on the skin overlying the cartilage tissue such as the nose and ears

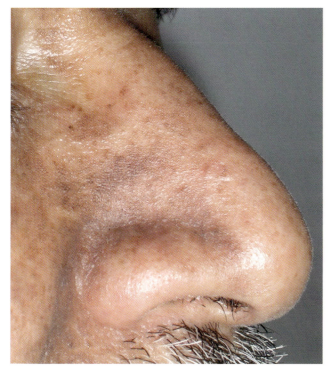

Fig. 1.1. Drug-induced hyperpigmentation

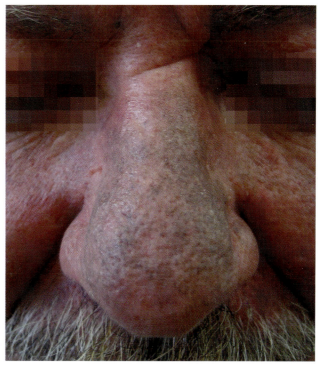

Fig. 1.2. PUVA therapy-induced hyperpigmentation

(Fig. 1.3). Arthropathy and intervertebral disc calcification are the major systemic findings, and cardiac involvement may cause myocardial infarction. The patient's urine typically turns dark after it is left at room temperature. Argyria is caused by the deposition of silver particles in the skin and mucosal surfaces. The prolonged use of nose drops containing silver can cause a slate-grey pigmentation on the nose and face. Local discolouration can also occur after the excessive use of silver sulfadiazine containing creams for burns. Actinic lichen planus is a clinical variant of lichen planus that typically affects the sun-exposed areas like the nose, producing brown to black patches or flat plaques with irregular borders. Lichen planus pigmentosus may also involve the face and nose as brown or greyish black macules (Fig. 1.4). Acanthosis nigricans, which is often seen in flexural areas, can also present with hyperpigmentation on ala nasi. Severe forms and atypically located lesions can be associated with malignancies.

Ephelides (freckles) are common pigmented lesions of the nose and cheeks which are often seen in early childhood (Fig. 1.5). The patients are usually fair-skinned and have blue or green eyes. The tan-brown irregular, small macules become prominent in summer. Lentigo can also be located on the nose. The nose is mostly covered with lentigines and ephelides in xeroderma pigmentosum (Fig. 1.6). The early (in situ) lesions of lentigo malignant melanoma are called "lentigo maligna" which present with irregular hyperpigmented macules on the nose (Fig. 1.7, 1.8). Mostly related to chronic sun exposure, the lesions become elevated as the tumor progresses into the invasive stage. Early diagnosis is important for effective treatment. The early lesions of seborrheic keratosis, pigmented actinic keratosis and lentigo solaris can resemble lentigo maligna. Blue or bluish grey, usually unilateral pigmentation located on the skin and mucosal surfaces supplied by the first and second branches of the trigeminal nerve is seen in nevus of Ota (Fig. 1.9). Eyelids, forehead, temple, nasal root and ala nasi can be affected by this dermal melanocytic tumor. Bluish grey pigmentation of the sclera

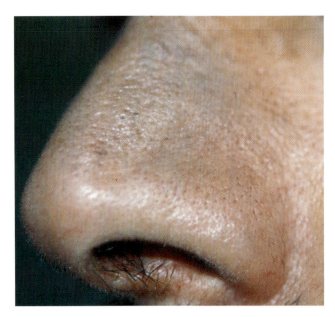

Fig. 1.3. Ochronosis

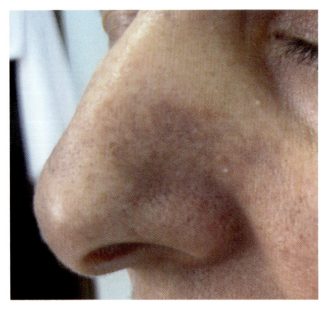

Fig. 1.4. Lichen planus pigmentosus

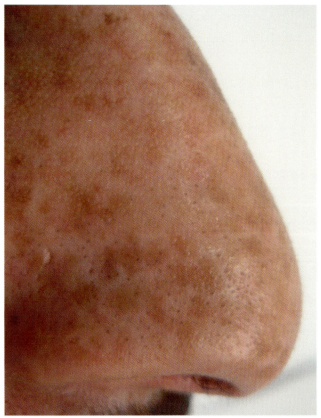

Fig. 1.5. Ephelides

1 Macular Lesions

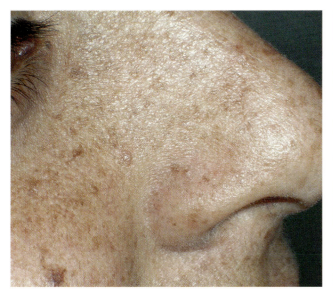

Fig. 1.6. Xeroderma pigmentosum

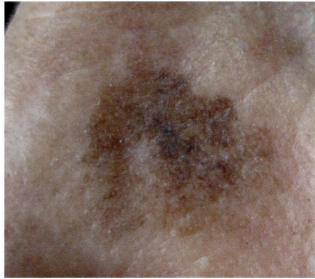

Fig. 1.8. Lentigo malignant melanoma. In situ stage

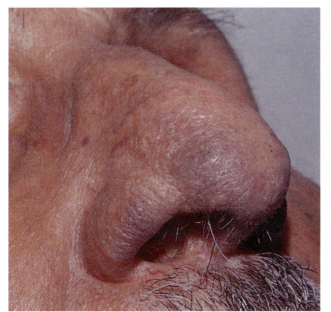

Fig. 1.7. Lentigo malignant melanoma. In situ stage

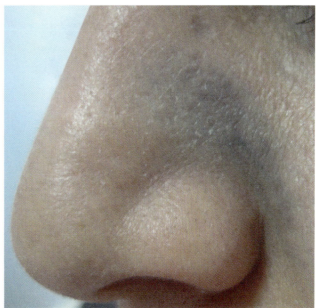

Fig. 1.9. Nevus of Ota

may be prominent in some patients. Pigmentation can also be seen in the nasal mucosa. Rarely, malignant melanoma can develop on the macular skin lesions. Therefore the patients must be followed up regularly.

The hypopigmented macules on the nose are usually caused by vitiligo (Fig. 1.10). Although this common pigmentation disorder can affect different parts of the body, facial lesions of vitiligo often cause a more serious cosmetic problem. Piebaldism is a rare congenital localized pigmentary disorder that mostly involves the forehead and scalp in the midline producing a white forelock. The hypopigmented macule can affect vertex and the nose. Patches of hyperpigmentation can be seen within and in the border of white mac-

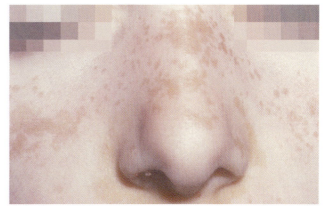

Fig. 1.10. Vitiligo

ules. Pityriasis alba can also cause hypopigmented macules with fine scales that are round or annular in shape and mostly 1-2 cm in size. It is commonly seen in children and spontaneously disappears after a few years. Postinflammatory hypopigmentation (Fig. 1.11) or hyperpigmentation can occur as a result of surgical procedures performed for the common tumors of this region and also after radiotherapy. Plaques of discoid lupus erythematosus may also leave hypo- (Fig. 1.12) or hyperpigmentation after they resolve.

Erythema, purpura and angiomatous lesions can present with red macules. Erythema can disappear spontaneously after a short period of time or persist in some diseases. The malar rash in systemic lupus erythematosus (SLE) is noticed on both cheeks and nasal bridge as persistent, asymptomatic erythema (Fig. 1.13). It can present in different forms other than the classical "butterfly" pattern, and often accompanies the systemic findings of the disease. The course of skin change is unpredictable in SLE. Generally, skin flares coincide with systemic flares. Rosacea begins with flushing, and later a persistent erythema occurs on the midface (Fig. 1.14). This chronic disease is more commonly seen in middle-aged women. While erythema on the nose can be the only manifestation, pink hemispherical papules, pustules and telangiectases can also be observed. Sometimes erythema shows a "butterfly" pattern similar to SLE. But, systemic symptoms do not accompany rosacea. Perioral dermatitis, which usually occurs after the prolonged use of topical corticosteroids, can also cause erythema or small papulopustular lesions on the nose in addition to the typical perioral lesions.

Facial erythema can develop in early childhood period in some genodermatoses that are related with photosensitivity. The erythema prominently involving the cheeks, nose and forehead starts in the first 3-6 months of life and soon evolves into poikilodermatous changes in Rothmund-Thom-

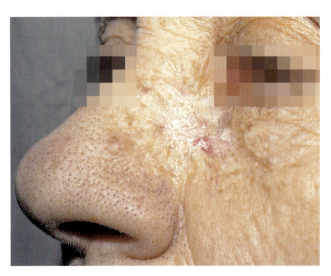

Fig. 1.11. Radiodermatitis. Postinflammatory hypopigmentation

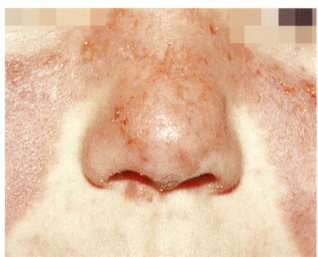

Fig. 1.13. Systemic lupus erythematosus. Malar rash

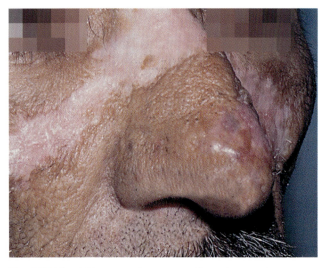

Fig. 1.12. Discoid lupus erythematosus. Hypopigmentation

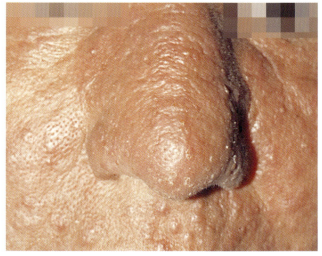

Fig. 1.14. Rosacea

son syndrome (Fig. 1.15). Erythema on the cheeks usually appear within the first month of life in Bloom's syndrome which is a congenital disorder associated with photosensitivity, dwarfism, hypogonadism and increased incidence of malignancies such as leukemia, lymphoma, Wilms' tumor and gastrointestinal carcinomas. Telangiectases develop on persistent erythema that spreads to involve other parts of the face like the nose, forehead, and ears, extensor surfaces of the arms and dorsum of the hands leading to poikiloderma. Cutaneous malignancies are rarely reported, probably due to the reduced life expectancy. The initial cutaneous finding of erythropoietic protoporphyria can be a "butterfly" rash occuring in early childhood due to extreme photosensitivity that accompanies edema and burning sensation. Life-long avoidance of sun exposure is essential in disorders of photosensitivity.

Erysipelas and cellulitis are common acute infections that affect the face. They are caused mostly by Streptococcus pyogenes and occasionally other organisms. The bacteria can enter the skin in the setting of other infections like folliculitis and herpes simplex, or abrasions and ulcers that alter the skin barrier (Fig. 1.16). Patients are usually adults. Erythema often starts suddenly on the nasal bridge. It may be limited to the nose or spread to the cheeks. The lesions of erysipelas are relatively more elevated than cellulitis. Systemic findings like pyrexia and chills support the diagnosis. Response to systemic antibiotics is fast in both infections. Cellulitis sometimes shows a recurrent course on the nose. Acrodynia (pink disease) is a form of mercury poisoning that typically occurs in infants or young children. The nose may be pink together with the hands being red. Photophobia, excessive sweating, excessive secretion of saliva, loss of appetite, hypertension, pruritus, cold painful hands and feet are other findings of this rare disease. Purpura may frequently be caused by mechanical trauma on the nose.

Congenital or acquired angiomatous macules can be seen on the nose. The macular lesions of port-wine-stain type of nevus flammeus are usually unilateral on the face extending from the side of the nose to adjacent cheek and forehead. The lesions are sharply-marginated with pink to red colouration at birth which change to purple within years (Fig. 1.17). In

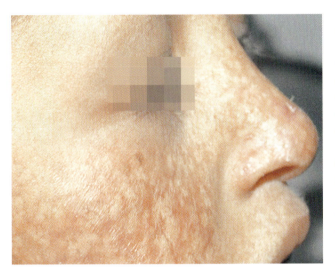

Fig. 1.15. Rothmund-Thomson syndrome

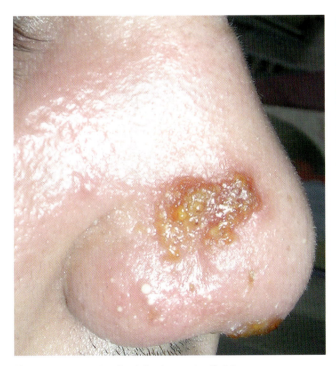

Fig. 1.16. Herpes simplex infection and cellulitis

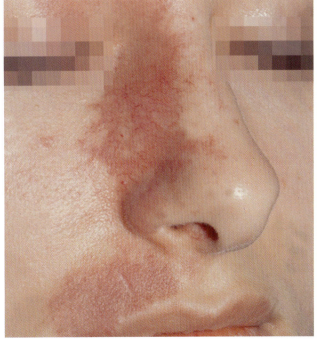

Fig. 1.17. Nevus flammeus. Port-wine-stain

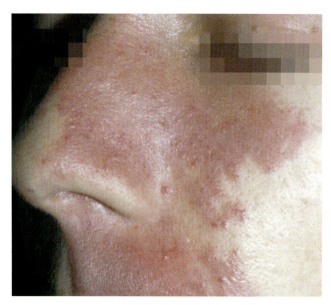

Fig. 1.18. Sturge-Weber syndrome. Nevus flammeus

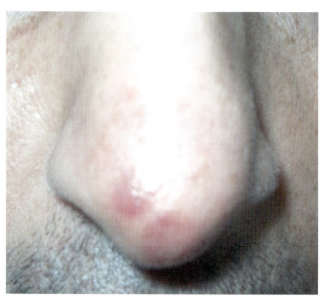

Fig. 1.20. Kaposi's sarcoma

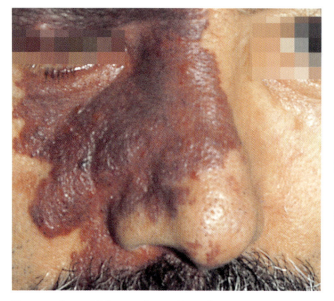

Fig. 1.19. Sturge-Weber syndrome. Nevus flammeus

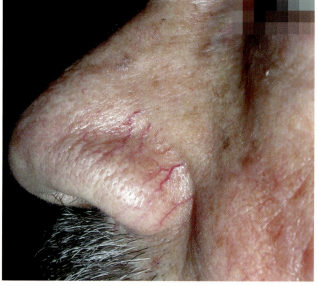

Fig. 1.21. Idiopathic telangiectasia

Sturge-Weber syndrome the angiomas are particularly located on the distribution of the sensory innervation of the first and second branches of the trigeminal nerve (Fig. 1.18). The patients must be carefully checked for intracranial calcification and glaucoma. Some patients are otherwise healthy. The macular lesions of port-wine-stain may become infiltrated and show surface irregularities in adulthood (Fig. 1.19). On the other hand, the pink macules of salmon patch type of nevus flammeus involving the nose at birth mostly resolve spontaneously. The early stages of Kaposi's sarcoma can present with pink, red to brown or purple angiomatous macules on the nose (Fig. 1.20). Lesions on this region are more commonly seen in HIV infected patients. The early lesions of angiosarcoma, especially seen after middle age, can be ecchymotic macules on the midface that have irregular borders.

Telangiectases are commonly seen on the nose of adults. They are usually located on ala nasi as short red streaks that are at skin level or mildly elevated (Fig. 1.21). They are not related to rosacea or any systemic diseases if there are no accompanying cutaneous lesions. Chronic ultraviolet light

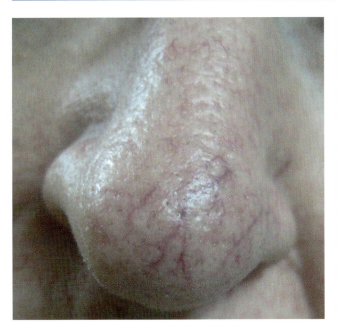

Fig. 1.22. Chronic ultraviolet light damage. Telangiectasia

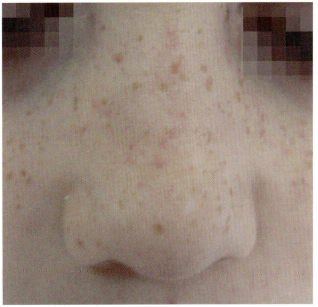

Fig. 1.24. Rendu-Osler-Weber syndrome. Telangiectasia

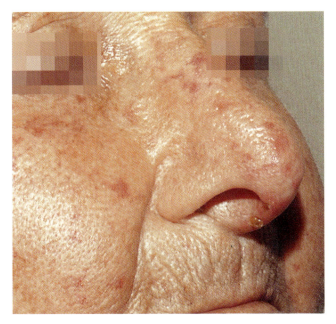

Fig. 1.23. CREST syndrome. Telangiectasia

damage (Fig. 1.22) especially in fair-skinned individuals, prolonged use of topical corticosteroids and rhinoplasty can also cause telangiectasia. The nose may appear red in cases of dense telangiectases. The nose can be covered with telangiectases in CREST syndrome and Rendu-Osler-Weber syndrome. CREST syndrome is a form of scleroderma that is localized to acral regions and face with dense calcification and prominent telangiectases especially on the face and palms (Fig. 1.23). Rendu-Osler-Weber syndrome (hereditary hemorrhagic telangiectasia) can present with telangiectases on different parts of the body including the face starting from puberty (Fig. 1.24). Telangiectases of the lips and tongue can also be seen in this genodermatosis. Telangiectases in the nose frequently bleed and cause iron deficiency anemia.

Palmoplantar keratoderma, sclerodactyly, scleroatrophy and nail dystrophy are characteristics of Huriez syndrome that is also associated with telangiectases on the lips and poikiloderma-like changes on the nose. The patients have a high risk of developing squamous cell carcinoma on the affected skin in adulthood.

2 ■ Vesiculobullous and Pustular Lesions

While vesiculous, bullous and pustular elementary lesions can be seen in different diseases, vesicles and bullae (blisters) can also transform into pustules over time. The difference between vesicles and bullae depends only on the size. Hence, these three elementary lesions can be seen together in the same disease. Viral and bacterial infections, immunobullous dermatoses and photodermatoses are the major diseases that present with vesicles, bullae and pustules on the nose. On the other hand, papules and vesicles can rarely be seen together in some diseases.

Granulosis rubra nasi consists of papules and vesicles that are limited to the nose. This disease is mostly seen before puberty. Papules and sometimes vesicles can be seen on the tip of the nose which usually seems wet because of regional excessive sweating (Fig. 2.1, 2.2). Persistent erythema and purplish colour can appear over time. Patients may complain of pruritus and burning sensation. The relationship between systemic diseases and this idiopathic dermatosis is not defined. Lesions persist for many years and disappear completely during puberty.

Herpes simplex infection caused by *HSV-1* is typically seen on the face around the mouth and nose. Group of vesicles appear on a background of erythema on the tip of the nose and ala nasi, develop into pustules and often crust in a few days during the course of recurrent attacks of the infection (Fig. 2.3). Lesions usually heal within a few days without scarring. On the other hand, primary herpes simplex infection which is more severe and cause systemic symptoms can also be seen on the tip of the nose. Vesiculopustular lesions of varicella (chicken pox) typically involve the scalp

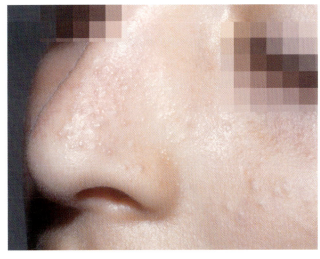

Fig. 2.2. Granulosis rubra nasi

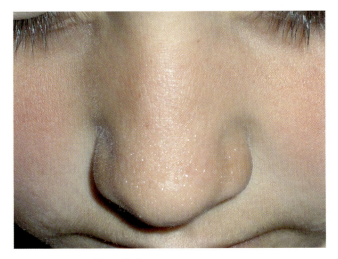

Fig. 2.1. Regional hyperhidrosis

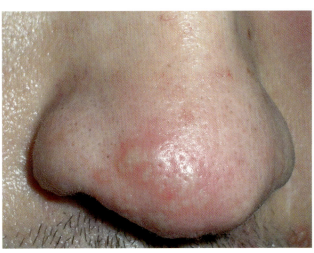

Fig. 2.3. Herpes simplex infection

and the face, so these pruritic lesions can be prominent on the nose (Fig. 2.4). Ophthalmic zoster, resulting from the reactivation of *Varicella zoster virus,* involves the first branch of the trigeminal nerve causing unilateral vesicles on the eyelid, forehead and in front of the scalp. Ocular involvement should be suspected when blisters are seen unilaterally on the nose, indicating involvement of the nasocilliary branch (Hutchinson sign) (Fig. 2.5). Afterwards, vesicles become purulent and develop into necrotic crusts and ulcers. Patients usually suffer from intense pain. Lesions may last longer when compared with herpes zoster lesions of the trunk. Systemic antiviral therapy is indicated to prevent the complications like uveitis and keratitis. Post-herpetic neuralgia is a frequent problem in patients with ophthalmic zoster.

Impetigo, a superficial bacterial infection, develops on the nose usually after long lasting flu infection. It is most common among children (Fig. 2.6). Clinically it can be seen as bullous and nonbullous impetigo (impetigo contagiosa). Usually *Staphylococcus aureus* is responsible for the bullous form and Streptococcus sp. for the nonbullous form, however this distinction is currently not considered important. As S. aureus colonizes the nasal mucosa, the infection may start in the perinasal area in carriers of the bacteria and spread to the periphery. Blisters typically rupture and leave characteristic honey-coloured crusts. Perinasal crusting and serum leakage are commonly observed presentations (Fig. 2.7). The infection responds well to antibiotic therapy and all lesions heal without scarring. Staphylococcal folliculitis is usually seen

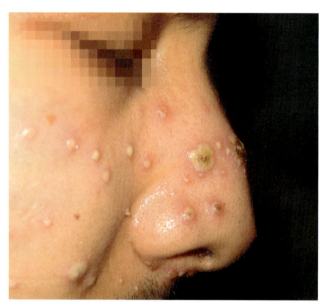

Fig. 2.4. Varicella

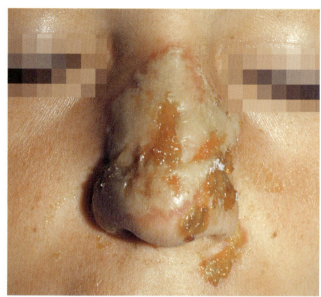

Fig. 2.6. Impetigo

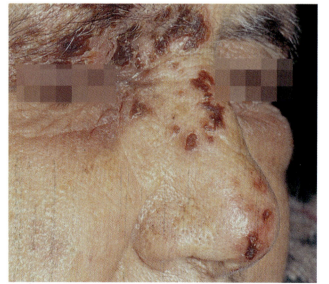

Fig. 2.5. Ophtalmic zoster

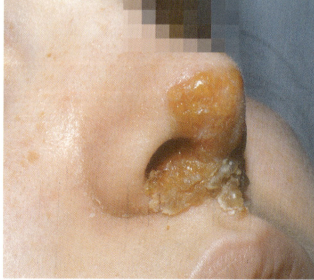

Fig. 2.7. Impetigo

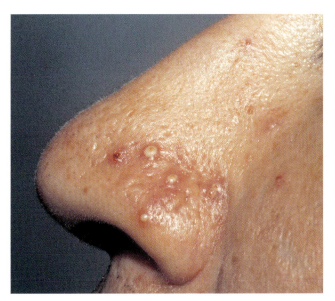

Fig. 2.8. Staphyloccal folliculitis

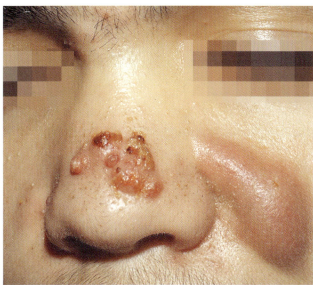

Fig. 2.10. Acne vulgaris

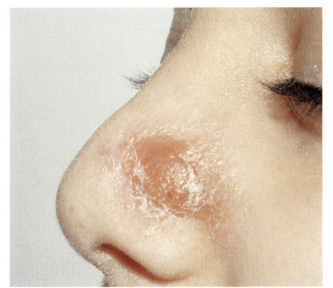

Fig. 2.9. Furuncle

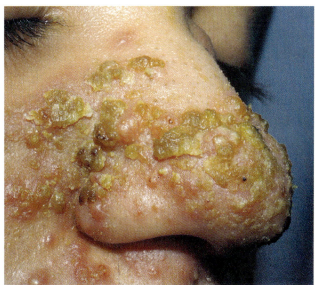

Fig. 2.11. Acne vulgaris. Secondary impetiginization

on the ala nasi as superficial pustules (Fig. 2.8). Another staphylococcal infection, furuncle, presents with a deeply located inflammatory nodule with a central pustule (Fig. 2.9). Although low, there is a risk of development of cavernous sinus thrombosis after pyodermas on the nose, therefore treatment with systemic antibiotics is necessary.

Cat scratch disease, which starts as a papule or a crusted pustule at the site of inoculation after being scratched by a cat, is a chronic infection caused by a gram negative bacillus, called *Bartonella henselae.* Abscess like lesions usually involving the tip of the nose, can be observed. It is one of the most common causes of lymphadenopathy lasting more than 3-4 weeks, in childhood and puberty. This infection usually regresses spontaneously. Acne vulgaris is commonly seen on the nose where the hair follicles are dense and the secretion of seborrheic glands is increased. Lesions also involve other parts of the face and sometimes the ears. Inflammatory papules, pustules, cysts and comedones can frequently be observed together (Fig. 2.10). Some pustules may impetiginize and be crusted (Fig. 2.11), and cystic lesions may rarely develop into abscesses. *Demodex folliculorum* mites are located in the hair follicles, and under some conditions they may be pathogenic causing demodicosis. Nose is one of the typical sites of demodicosis because of excessive production of sebum which is used as food by the mites. A rosacea-like appearance with follicular papules and superficial pustules are observed, especially when the immune system is suppressed. Epidermal growth factor receptor (EGFR)

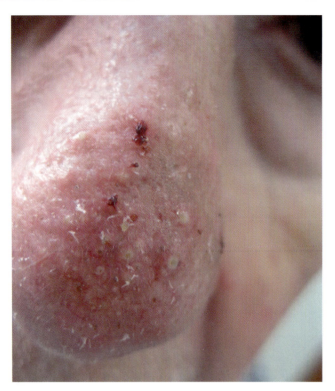

Fig. 2.12. Epidermal growth factor receptor antogonists-induced drug eruption

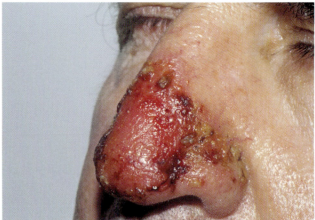

Fig. 2.14. Pemphigus vulgaris

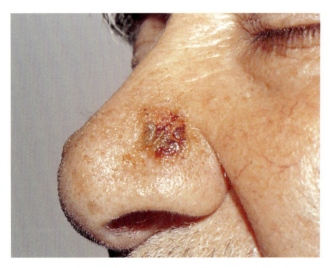

Fig. 2.13. Pemphigus vulgaris

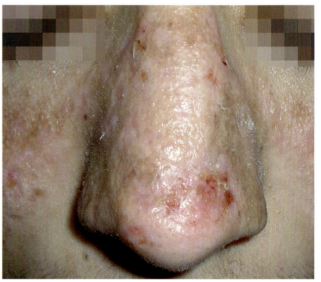

Fig. 2.15. Hydroa vacciniforme

antogonists-induced drug eruption may present with pustules on the face, especially on the nose (Fig. 2.12).

Pemphigus vulgaris should be suspected when there are non-healing erosions and crusts on the nose (Fig. 2.13, 2.14). Intact flaccid blisters are not common in this area. These erosions are usually located on the ala nasi uni- or bilaterally and can even cover the entire nose. Although rare, it must be remembered that pemphigus vulgaris may be restricted to the nose and may relapse after therapy at the same site. In some cases pemphigus vulgaris may involve the nasal mucosa causing chronic erosions, crusting and sometimes nasal congestion, discharge or epistaxis. Bullous pemphigoid may occasionally be seen on the nose both with intact bullae and erosions. Linear IgA dermatosis may present with tense nasal bullae on an erythematous base in adults. Similar lesions may be seen in chronic bullous dermatosis of childhood around the ages of 4 and 5. Bullae on other parts of the body mostly accompany nasal lesions in both diseases. Patients may complain of pruritus and burning sensation. Erosive and crusted lesions may be encountered on the cheeks, eyelids and nose in patients with Stevens-Johnson syndrome, a severe form of erythema multiforme which is usually caused by medications. Oral mucosal involvement with crusting on the lips is commonly observed in these patients.

Hydroa vacciniforme is a type of photodermatosis seen in childhood. It causes recurrent crops of umbilicated, tiny vesicles on the nose and cheeks which evolve into hemorrhagic, necrotic or crusted lesions. They resolve typically

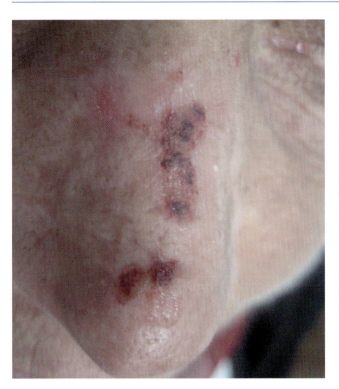

Fig. 2.16. Porphyria cutanea tarda

with variola-like scars (Fig. 2.15). Actinic prurigo is another photodermatosis affecting the face. It is more commonly seen in girls at 8 to 14 years of age. They may also have family history. Papules and vesicles which tend to eczematize over time are observed on sun-exposed areas like nose, cheeks, forehead and ears. Porphyria cutanea tarda, the most common form of porphyrias, involves sun-exposed areas causing bullae, erosions, crusts, dyspigmentation and atrophic scars on the nose (Fig. 2.16). Since acute photosensitivity is rarely seen, patients may deny the role of the sun. Milia, large comedones and hypertrichosis may also be observed on the face in the course of the disease. In congenital erythropoietic porphyria (Günther's disease) there may be atrophic scars on the nose due to recurrent vesiculobullous lesions. These may be present since birth or develop secondary to infections. In addition, severe photosensitivity and growth retardation are seen in these children. The diagnostic clinical feature of the disease is erythrodontia of both the primary and permanent teeth.

3 ■ Eczematous and Squamous Lesions

Eczematous lesions, namely erythematous, scaly (squamous), crusted and sometimes oozing lesions are not only seen in contact dermatitis, but also in other diseases with different etiologies. In some diseases scales are more prominent. The superficial types of pemphigus including pemphigus foliaceus (Fig. 3.1) and pemphigus seborrheicus (Fig. 3.2) may present with eczematous patches on the nose. These lesions are more commonly observed in adult patients. While pemphigus foliaceus often causes disseminated lesions, pemphigus seborrheicus presents with localized ones. In these entities, intact bullae are not usually present. Instead, scales and crusts on an erythematous base intermingled with small eroded areas are commonly observed. Therefore, some patients may be misdiagnosed and mistreated as contact dermatitis for a long time. Pemphigus seborrheicus may sometimes resemble systemic lupus erythematosus due to symmetrical involvement, seen on the cheeks and nose in a butterfly-like pattern. Mucosal involvement is rare and response to treatment is better when compared to pemphigus vulgaris. On the other hand, some of the untreated pemphigus vulgaris lesions located on the nose may also become eczematized over time (Fig. 3.3).

Compared to the other parts of the face, contact dermatitis (eczema) localized to the nose seems to be rare. Irritant contact dermatitis may occur in the perinasal area due to frequent nose wiping during flu (Fig. 3.4). It may also be seen during topical treatment of nasal actinic keratoses with 5-fluorouracil and imiquimod. Inhalation of volatile solvents may cause perinasal irritant dermatitis. Irritant or allergic eczematous contact dermatitis may be observed on the root of the nose due to contact with the frame of glasses. Involvement of nasal skin may be observed as a result of the dissemination of allergic eczematous contact dermatitis starting from other parts of the face like cheeks and eyelids. In the acute phase of allergic eczema erythema, edema, blisters, weeping and crusts are seen while the chronic lesions are mostly dry, scaly and lichenified (Fig. 3.5).

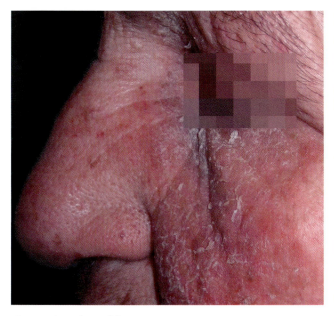

Fig. 3.1. Pemphigus foliaceus

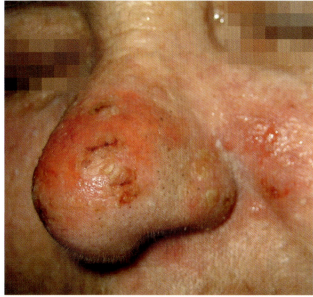

Fig. 3.2. Pemphigus seborrheicus

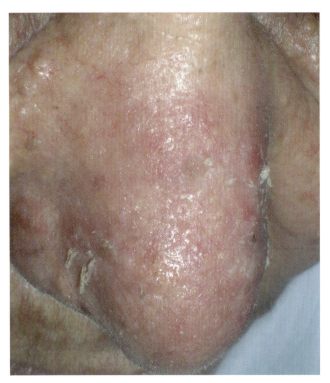

Fig. 3.3. Pemphigus vulgaris

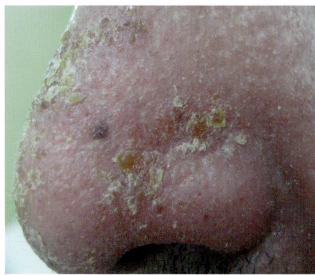

Fig. 3.5. Allergic eczematous contact dermatitis

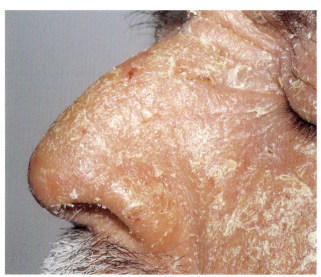

Fig. 3.6. Photoallergic drug reaction

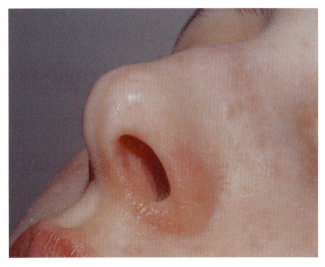

Fig. 3.4. Irritant contact dermatitis

Phototoxic and photoallergic drug reactions may involve the nose as well as other parts of the face (Fig. 3.6). History of drug use concomitant with sun exposure before the outbreak of the eczematous lesions is typical in these patients.

An eczematous eruption on photosensitive areas of the body may also be observed in pellagra that develops as a result of nicotinic acid or tryptophan deficiency and involves the gastrointestinal system, central nervous system and skin. The bridge of the nose is erythematous, and fine, yellow-coloured scales are observed on the follicular openings. Patients may complain of a burning sensation. The lesions regress rapidly after the treatment of the vitamin deficiency.

Seborrheic dermatitis may be observed in adults as bilateral, mostly ill-defined, pink-coloured patches with fine, loose scales localized on ala nasi and nasolabial folds. In some cases accumulation of yellow, thick scales or crusts can be seen on the entire nose (Fig. 3.7, 3.8). The symmetrical involvement of the nasal bridge and cheeks may cause a "butterfly appearance" similar to the malar rash of systemic lupus erythematosus. While some lesions may be sharply-defined, some are fissurized and crusted. Scalp involvement is seen in most of the patients. Seborrheic dermatitis may not cause

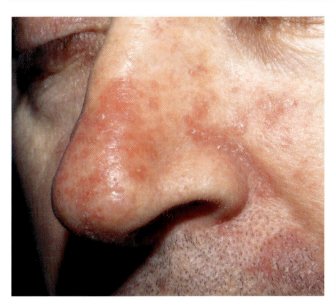
Fig. 3.7. Seborrheic dermatitis

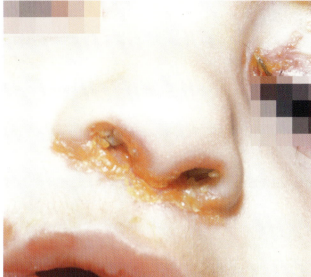
Fig. 3.9. Acrodermatitis enteropathica

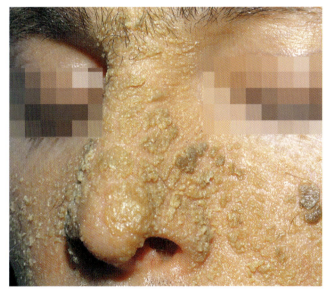
Fig. 3.8. Seborrheic dermatitis

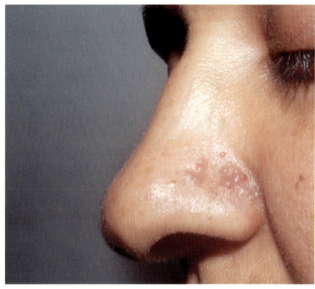
Fig. 3.10. Langerhans cell histiocytosis

pruritus even if severe. This condition responses well to treatment, but usually relapses at the same area just after stopping medication and shows a chronic course. Seborrheic dermatitis is very common in patients with AIDS, and dissemination with severe inflammation can be seen in these patients.

Acrodermatitis enteropathica is a disorder of zinc absorption with cutaneous and gastrointestinal involvement seen in infancy. It typically involves acral and periorificial regions. It may cause eczematous or psoriasiform plaques around nares (Fig. 3.9). Alopecia and severe diarrhea are other common symptoms of this disease. Zinc replacement leads to rapid improvement of the symptoms. A similar clinical picture could be seen in adults as a result of deficient zinc intake. In Langerhans cell histiocytosis, eczematous and sometimes purpuric lesions are most commonly seen on the flexural areas and scalp. Though not very common, nasal involvement may also be seen in this entity (Fig. 3.10). Most patients are children, but adults can also be affected. Papulonodular or ulcerated lesions can be seen in addition to petechiae, weeping and eczematization. Skin lesions have a chronic relapsing course. Erosions and ulcers can occur in oral and genital mucosal surfaces. Systemic involvement determines the prognosis of this disease.

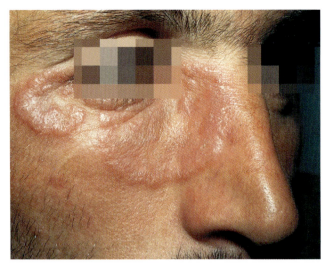

Fig. 3.11. Tinea faciei

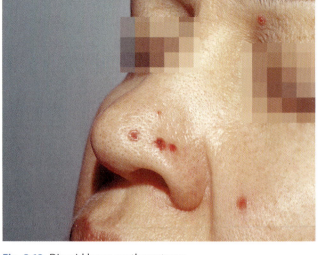

Fig. 3.13. Discoid lupus erythematosus

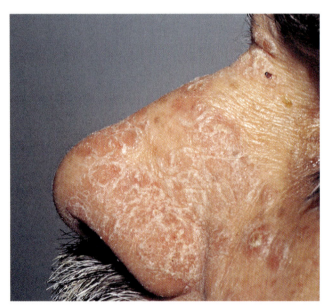

Fig. 3.12. Psoriasis vulgaris

Fig. 3.14. Discoid lupus erythematosus

Tinea faciei presents with sharply marginated, erythematous, scaly and dry plaques on the face. An asymmetrical distribution is seen in most cases. It can be hard to diagnose this fungal infection when only the nose is affected. The older central part of the annular or polycyclic plaque has a tendency to resolve and the peripheral part slowly enlarges. The border is inflammatory, red and scaly (Fig. 3.11). But these typical features may not be observed in all cases. Incorrect treatment with corticosteroids may cause the disappearance of the well-defined border. The severity of pruritus varies significantly between individual patients. The dermatophytes can rapidly be identified with KOH examination (native preparation). Sometimes culture can be used to identify the species. The lesions regress with topical antifungal therapy without scarring. Resistant or disseminated lesions need to be treated with systemic antifungal therapy.

Psoriasis vulgaris rarely affects the face and nose. However, psoriasis must be considered in the differential diagnosis of erythematous, squamous and dry plaques occuring in any part of the body (Fig. 3.12). The patients can be of any age and most have involvement of other regions. Discoid lupus erythematosus, which is clearly related with ultraviolet light exposure, is commonly seen on the nose of adult patients. Well-defined, erythematous, annular or oval plaques sometimes with adherent scales, have a predilection for the bridge of the nose (Fig. 3.13, 3.14). The lesions sometimes localize around the nares and can extend to the mucosa (Fig. 3.15).

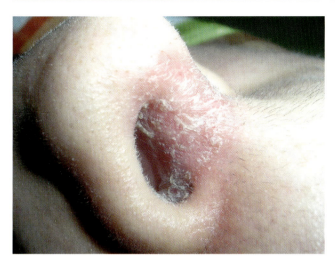 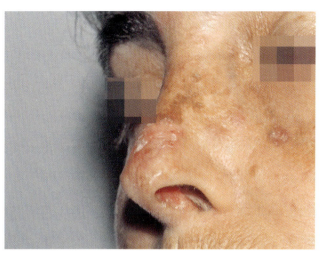

Fig. 3.15. Discoid lupus erythematosus

Fig. 3.16. Mixed connective tissue disorder

The patients with discoid lupus erythematosus may present with multiple lesions on the nose, ears and other parts of the body. Systemic lupus erythematosus does not accompany in most of the cases. The disease has a chronic relapsing course and recurrences are typically seen when the patients fail to protect themselves against ultraviolet light. The typical beaked nose appearance due to sclerodermatous changes may be observed in mixed connective tissue disorder besides the skin lesions of lupus erythematosus (Fig. 3.16).

4 ■ Hyperkeratotic Lesions

Hyperkeratosis, the thickening of the stratum corneum, is not common on the nose but it can be particularly seen in diseases that present with acral keratosis, genodermatoses, precancerous lesions and warts. A paraneoplastic disease, acrokeratosis paraneoplastica (Bazex syndrome), presents with acquired keratosis of the nasal tip and other acral areas that accompany solid malignancies of upper airways and the gastrointestinal system. Men are more commonly affected. Metastatic disease may have already been diagnosed at the time of skin presentation. Mild ichthyosiform changes on the body and sharply demarcated hyperkeratosis on the nose occur in KID syndrome, a genodermatosis associated with keratitis and deafness (Fig. 4.1). Alopecia and palmoplantar hyperkeratosis are present in most of the patients. Darier's disease is a keratinization disorder which has a predilection for seborrheic areas. Persistent greasy hyperkeratotic small papules may sometimes cover the entire nasal surface in these patients (Fig. 4.2).

Porokeratosis is a keratinization disorder which may be occasionally seen on the nose with irregularly-shaped plaques that are horny at the periphery and slightly atrophic at the centre (Fig. 4.3). Most of these lesions are superficial, but they may

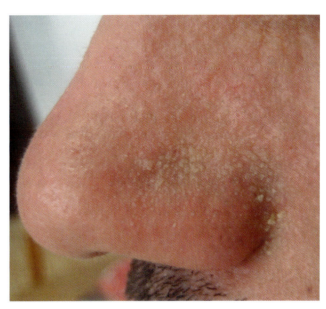

Fig. 4.2. Darier's disease

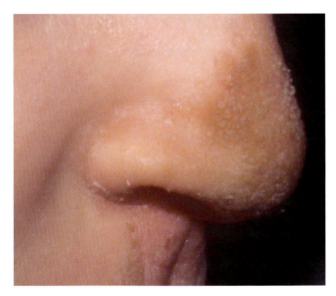

Fig. 4.1. KID syndrome

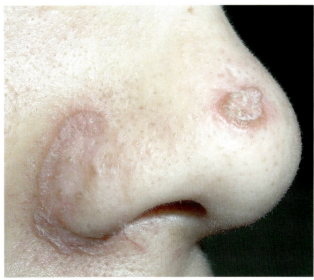

Fig. 4.3. Porokeratosis

rarely be destructive. Small flat plaques of actinic keratosis with adherent yellow- or brown-coloured scales can frequently be observed on the nose (Fig. 4.4). This disease is common among fair-tanned adults who have been exposed to sunlight for a long period of time. The rough surface of the early lesions is best identified by palpation rather than inspection. Although rare, the untreated lesions of actinic keratosis may evolve into squamous cell carcinoma. Protection against sunlight is the mainstay of the management, which also prevents the occurrence of new lesions. Verruca vulgaris is caused by various strains of the *Human papilloma virus* (HPV). It is commonly observed on the nose, either on the skin or on the vestibule (Fig. 4.5). Filiform verrucae are characterized with long, thin, filiform protuberances common on the nasal tip and around the nares (Fig. 4.6). Sometimes the papulonodular lesions of verrucae can cover the entire skin around nares (Fig. 4.7). Nasal cocaine abuse can cause verrucae in nasal mucosa. Inhalation tools which are shared among the cocaine users may act like a vector to spread the virus. The tools and cocaine crystals damage the mucosa, thus this region is more susceptible to viral infection. Cutaneous horn (cornu cutaneum) can be observed as a result of dense hyperkeratosis that occurs mostly on the basis of filliform warts as a conic-shaped eminence.

A late complication of radiotherapy applied to the skin tumors on the nose is chronic radiodermatitis which presents with poikilodermatous changes, sclerosis and hyperkeratosis

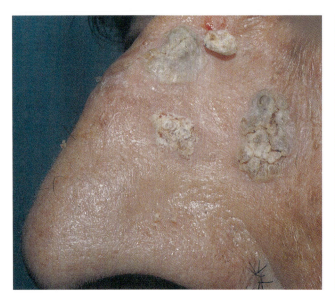

Fig. 4.4. Actinic keratosis

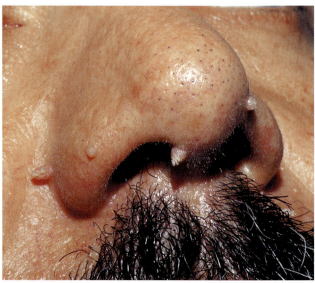

Fig. 4.6. Filiform verruca

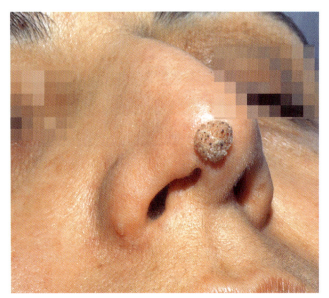

Fig. 4.5. Verruca vulgaris

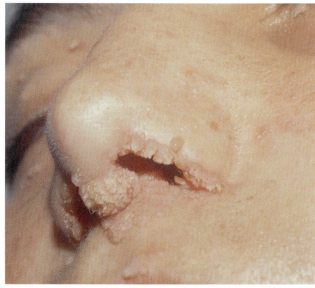

Fig. 4.7. Verruca vulgaris

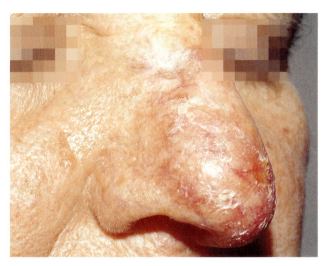

Fig. 4.8. Chronic radiodermatitis

on the nasal skin damaged by ionizing radiation (Fig. 4.8). Multiple myeloma patients can present with yellow-coloured spicules with horny appearance in the follicular openings of the face, particularly on the nose, rarely on the extremities, trunk and scalp. These spike-like, follicular hyperkeratotic lesions are reported to be eosinophilic deposits, that are cryoprecipitates composed of IgG-kappa with electrophoretic characteristics identical to those of the paraprotein present in the serum of the patient.

5 ■ Papular Lesions

Papules and nodules are two basic elementary lesions of the skin that are elevated but do not contain serum or pus; the difference between them depends only on the size. They can both be seen together in many diseases, however, one of them is usually more dominant. In this chapter, diseases that mostly present with papular (<1 cm) lesions will be discussed. Papules on the nose can frequently be observed due to many different causes, predominantly tumors and storage disorders. Some diseases are even named after the strict location of the lesions on the nose. Some of the benign tumoral lesions deserve special attention because they can be the initial sign of a systemic disease or a genodermatose. This relationship is more obvious when multiple papules are seen together. A similar scenario is also observed in basal cell carcinoma.

Fibrous papule of the nose is a flesh-coloured, 2-6 mm sized, dome-shaped papule mostly with a smooth surface. It is more commonly observed in middle age (Figs. 5.1, 5.2). This idiopathic benign lesion is mostly located on the tip of the nose or on the ala. While mostly solitary, there may sometimes be more than one lesion (Fig. 5.3). Rarely, it can be observed

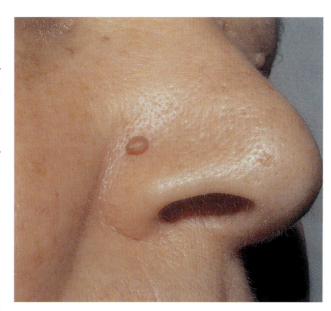

Fig. 5.2. Fibrous papule of the nose

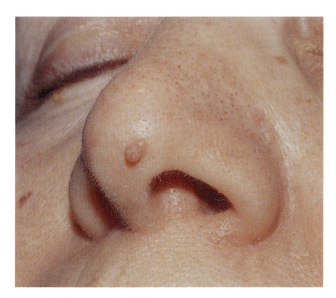

Fig. 5.1. Fibrous papule of the nose

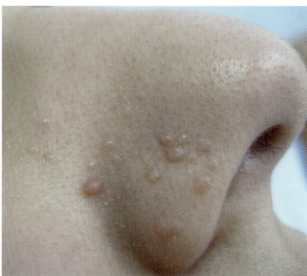

Fig. 5.3. Fibrous papule of the nose

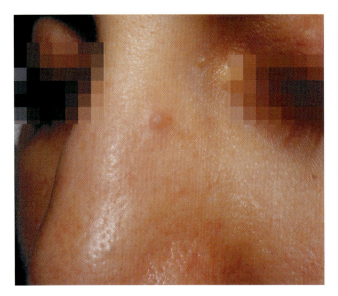

Fig. 5.4. Palisaded and encapsulated neuroma

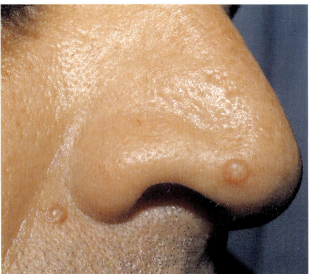

Fig. 5.5. Trichoepithelioma

on the neck and other parts of the face like cheeks and chin. Therefore it has also been named as fibrous papule of the face. It may sometimes be pedunculated. It only causes a cosmetic problem as patients do not have a subjective complaint. As the lesion does not have a risk of malignant transformation, therapy is not necessary. Palisaded and encapsulated neuroma is a benign nerve cell tumor that is mostly seen in middle age and is located on the nose and nasolabial folds (Fig. 5.4). It is a flesh- or pink-coloured solitary papule, 2-6 mm in size, and it may also be observed on other parts of the face. It is not associated with a systemic disease and there is no risk of malignant transformation. A rare hair follicle tumor, trichofolliculoma, can be seen on the nose as well as other areas of the face. The typical lesion is a flesh- or reddish-coloured, dome-shaped papule or nodule that bares a bunch of hair protruding from a central pore. It only poses a cosmetic problem.

Trichoepithelioma is a benign tumor of the hair follicle which may be observed as a solitary lesion on the nose in all ages starting from childhood (Fig. 5.5). It presents as a flesh- or pink-coloured, shiny papule with telangiectases on the surface. The lesion slowly enlarges, and the size can vary between 2 to 8 mm. It does not cause any symptoms. The solitary papules on the nose sometimes can only be differentiated with histopathologic examination. Idiopathic trichoepitheliomas are usually seen as a solitary papule or a few papules. Multiple lesions are referred as Brooke-Spiegler syndrome (epithelioma adenoides cysticum). These lesions mostly arise on the midface especially on the nose and nasolabial folds. Disseminated cylindromas which appear as larger nodules on different areas of the body may be observed in this familial disease. Grouped trichoepitheliomas on the nose can cause disfigurement (Fig. 5.6). Laser surgery is a therapeutic option when there are many lesions.

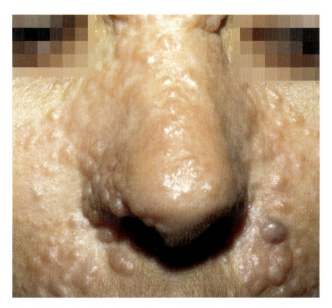

Fig. 5.6. Brooke-Spiegler syndrome. Multiple trichoepitheliomas

Perifollicular fibroma (fibrofolliculoma) is an acquired, 2-3 mm sized, flesh- or grey- to yellow-coloured, dome-shaped papule. This benign tumour of the fibrous root sheath of the hair follicle may be a solitary lesion or can be observed as many scattered papules on the face or neck (Fig. 5.7). When there are multiple lesions, a family history is usually present, and the lesions can be part of Birt-Hogg-Dubé syndrome (Fig. 5.8). Fibrofolliculoma, trichodiscoma and acrochordon are the benign tumors seen in this syndrome. Perifollicular fibroma, fibrofolliculoma, and trichodiscoma are considered to be part of the same clinicopathological spectrum. Though these tumours cause only a cosmetic problem, patients must

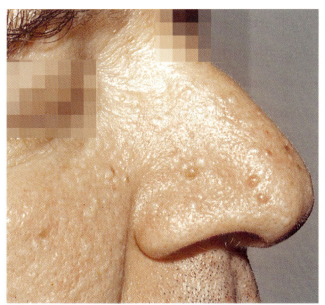

Fig. 5.7. Perifollicular fibroma

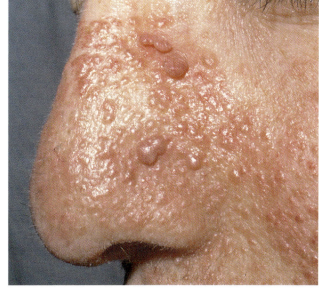

Fig. 5.9. Tuberous sclerosis. Angiofibroma

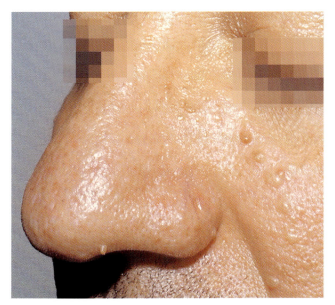

Fig. 5.8. Birt-Hogg-Dubé syndrome. Perifollicular fibroma

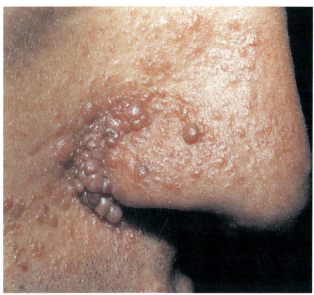

Fig. 5.10. Tuberous sclerosis. Angiofibroma

be screened for accompanying internal malignancies such as renal cell carcinoma, thyroid carcinoma and gastrointestinal carcinoma. Therefore a careful follow-up is recommended. Recurrent spontaneous pneumothorax is another feature of this syndrome. When a patient is diagnosed with Birt-Hogg-Dubé syndrome, the family must also be screened dermatologically and oncologically.

Tuberous sclerosis is another disease that presents with many small papules on the nose. Flesh-, pink- or reddish purple-coloured, dome-shaped, firm, 1 to 3 mm, symmetrically distributed papules on the nose and nasolabial folds are among the diagnostic features of this genodermatosis (Fig. 5.9). Facial papules occur between the ages of 2 to 6 years, and are angiofibromas histopathologically. They may cause a serious cosmetic problem over time when they increase in number. Hundreds of lesions may be seen sometimes. Papules may be grouped especially in nasolabial folds and ala nasi, and may transform into elevated nodules (Figs. 5.10, 5.11). Other dermatological features of tuberous sclerosis are benign tumors like collagen nevus, periungual fibroma, acrochordon and also hypopigmented macules. Systemic manifestations of the disease include central nervous system involvement presenting with infantile spasms, mental retardation and subependymal nodules, as well as retinal hamartomas, renal angiomyolipomas, cardiac rhabdomyomas and lymphangiomyomatosis of the lung.

Oral mucosal neuromas and cutaneous neuromas on the eyelids and nose which appear as small, pedunculated papules with smooth surface can be observed in MEN-2B syndrome. Medullary thyroid carcinoma and pheochromocytoma are the other features of this disease. Presence of neuromas is the pathognomonic sign which can alert one to a possible diagnosis of this syndrome and the need to screen for thyroid carcinoma. Many flesh- or yellow-coloured, 1-2 mm papules occur on the nose in Cowden syndrome (Fig. 5.12). Histopathologically these lesions are trichilemmomas, rare tumours of the outer root sheath of the hair follicle, and they are not limited to the nose. The diagnosis of this syndrome by skin lesions can lead to an early diagnosis of the accompanying malignancies like hamartomatous tumors of the breast and thyroid, and colonic polyps.

Translucent, gelatinous ear papules are the typical features of juvenile hyaline fibromatosis, but similar papules can also be observed on the nose (Fig. 5.13). Dermochondrocorneal dystrophy (François syndrome) presents with greyish to white-coloured, firm papulonodules symmetrically located on the dorsum of hands, nose and ears. Gingival and palatal mucosal hyperplasia may accompany. Osteochondrodystrophy of the hand and foot bones and white opacities on the cornea are other features of this genodermatosis, which has a slow but progressive course.

Eccrine hidrocystoma presents most commonly with multiple flesh- or bluish-coloured, translucent, 1-3 mm papules on the nose and cheeks. Characteristicly the papules enlarge in hot weather (Fig. 5.14). This benign eccrine gland tumor is not associated with a systemic disease. Milium is a tiny epidermoid cyst seen typically as yellow- or cream-coloured, 1-2 mm, firm papule on the cheeks, around the eyes and also on the nose. It commonly presents with multiple lesions. It may be idiopathic or can be observed in the course of some bullous dermatoses involving the dermoepidermal junction (Fig. 5.15). Senile sebaceous hyperplasia presents with yellow-coloured, soft, 2-5 mm papules with central umbilication on different parts of the face in adults (Fig. 5.16). These harmless lesions may be associated with cyclosporine use after transplantation. On the other hand, sebaceous gland hyperplasia can also be observed temporarily in newborns due to hormonal factors. They appear as yellow, tiny papules that are grouped on the ala nasi. Sebaceous gland hyperplasia on the nose may

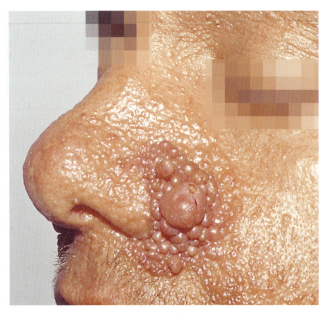

Fig. 5.11. Tuberous sclerosis. Angiofibroma

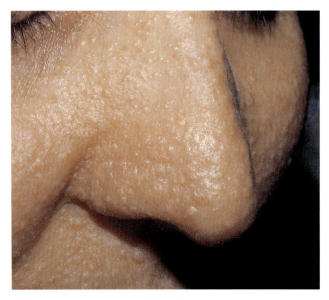

Fig. 5.12. Cowden syndrome. Trichilemmoma

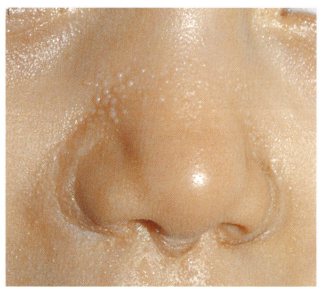

Fig. 5.13. Juvenile hyaline fibromatosis

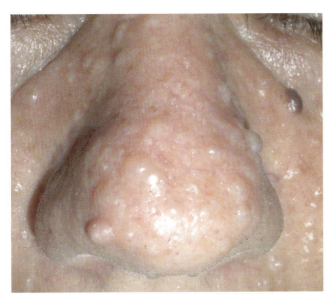

Fig. 5.14. Eccrine hidrocystoma

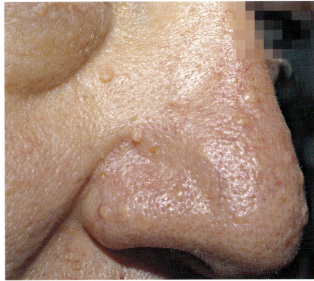

Fig. 5.16. Senile sebaceous hyperplasia

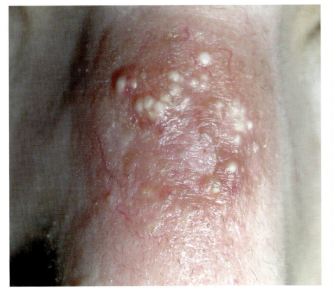

Fig. 5.15. Milia

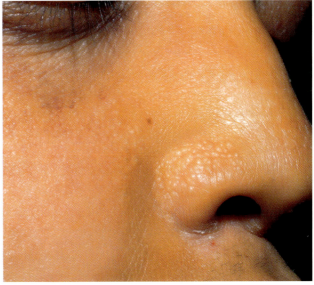

Fig. 5.17. Anhidrotic ectodermal dysplasia. Sebaceous gland hyperplasia

also be seen in anhidrotic ectodermal dysplasia in adulthood (Fig. 5.17). Syringoma is a benign eccrine gland tumor which present as multiple flat, flesh-coloured papules usually limited to the lower lids and cheeks. Sometimes it may also occur on the nose.

The most commonly observed malignant tumor of the skin, basal cell carcinoma, is primarily associated with chronic ultraviolet light damage, and is frequently located on the nose (Fig. 5.18). Typical initial lesion is a flesh- or pink-coloured, sometimes hyperpigmented papule with a smooth surface. While the tumor slowly enlarges, telangiectases appear on its surface and the centre depresses, thus its characteristic slightly elevated border becomes apparent. Gorlin syndrome (nevoid basal cell carcinoma syndrome) presents with multiple basal cell carcinomas that may be observed as small, flesh- or brown-coloured, dome-shaped papules on the nose and other parts of the face with an onset at childhood. These lesions may increase in number and enlarge later in adulthood, and may sometimes become ulcerated (Fig. 5.19). Milia, epidermoid cysts and palmoplantar pits are other cutaneous features of this disease. Besides, coarse facial appearance, odontogenic cysts of the jaws, fused ribs, calcification of falx cerebri, eye anomalies and ovarian fibromas can be observed in these patients. The differential diagnosis of Gorlin syndrome includes basaloid follicular hamartoma syndrome. This rare condition is characterized by hypothrichosis, hypohydrosis and palmoplantar pits which accompany the basaloid follicular hamartomas that have a predilection for the face, neck and scalp. These benign adnexal tumors consisting of basaloid cells with follicular differentiation are observed as skin-coloured or hyperpigmented papules. However, because this syndrome may be considered as a variant of Gorlin syndrome, patients must be followed up for development of malignancies. Bazex-Dupré-Christol syndrome can also present with multiple basal cell carcinomas on the nose and other parts of the face starting in the second or third decade. Hypotrichosis, milia, hypohidrosis and follicular atrophoderma are the accompanying dermatological features. Muir-Torre syndrome is associated with sebaceous adenomas which are observed as yellowish papules or nodules sometimes with verrucous surface that can be localized on the nose (Fig. 5.20). There is a high risk of development of gastrointestinal and genitourinary carcinomas in this syndrome. Therefore, when this sebaceous gland tumor is diagnosed, a detailed screening for internal malignancies must be carried out.

A rare type of non-Langerhans cell histiocytoses, xanthoma disseminatum, presents with yellow or brownish papules or nodules which are mostly located on flexural areas, but smooth surfaced papules can also be seen on the face, particularly on the nose (Fig. 5.21). Cutaneous lesions may

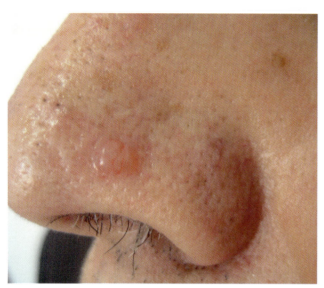

Fig. 5.18. Basal cell carcinoma

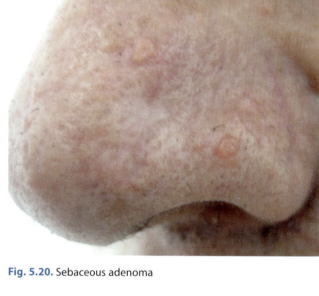

Fig. 5.20. Sebaceous adenoma

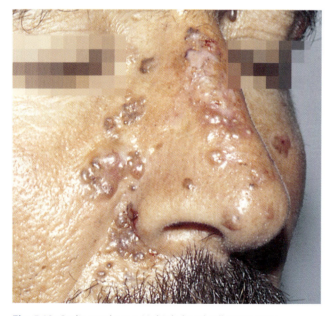

Fig. 5.19. Gorlin syndrome. Multiple basal cell carcinomas

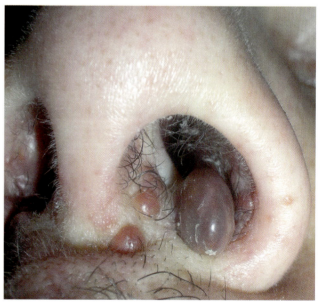

Fig. 5.21. Xanthoma disseminatum

enlarge into giant masses, and upper respiratory tract mucosal lesions can be life-threatening due to airway obstruction. Some patients have also diabetes insipidus. Brown to red papulonodular lesions on the face and sometimes on the nose can be observed in Rosai-Dorfman disease (massive lymphadenopathy with sinus histiocytosis). Cervical lymphadenopathy which makes the diagnosis easier may accompany the skin disease. When only skin lesions are present, the diagnosis is much harder. Sea blue histiocytosis is a rare progressive disease seen in childhood. Papulonodular lesions and elevated infiltrated plaques on the face and also on the nose are observed. The hands, feet and trunk may also be affected. Lung and liver involvement may be fatal. Langerhans cell histiocytosis (Hand-Schüller-Christian disease) presents with papulonodular lesions especially on flexural areas and causes an eruption similar to diffuse seborheic dermatitis. Lesions may sometimes be observed on the face and nose.

A congenital hamartomatous lesion, nevus sebaceus, can rarely be seen on the nose as coalescing papules forming plaques (Fig. 5.22). Spider angioma is a pulsatile, reddish papule, several millimeters in diameter, and has thin tortuous telangiectases radiating outwards from its center. It develops due to an arterial enlargement. The nose is a typical location (Figs. 5.23, 5.24). Solitary or only a few lesions usually occur in childhood or in early adulthood. It is mostly of idiopathic origin. Many and larger spider angiomas can be observed in hyperthyroidism, pregnancy, CREST syndrome and chronic liver failure. The lesions mostly cause a cosmetic problem, and can be treated with cauterization and laser. Pregnancy associated lesions may regress after birth. Senile angioma (cherry angioma) is a common benign tumor of adults presenting as multiple, small, red macules or smooth-surfaced papules mostly seen on the trunk. They are rarely located on the nose (Fig. 5.25). An association with systemic disease is not known for this type of capillary angioma.

Papules on the nose can be observed in some storage diseases. Grouped tiny papules on the face and sometimes on the nose can be seen in juvenile colloid milium (Fig. 5.26). Lignous periodontitis and lignous conjunctivitis are other features of the disease. Adult colloid milium is associated with solar damage and only involves the skin. It appears as many, soft, waxy, 1-5 mm sized papules seen mostly on cheeks, nose, ears and periorbital area. Gelatinous material can be drained from the lesions for diagnostic purposes. Papules do not have a tendency to resolve spontaneously. Flesh-coloured, dome-shaped or flat,

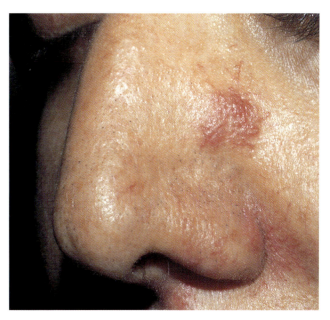

Fig. 5.23. Spider angioma

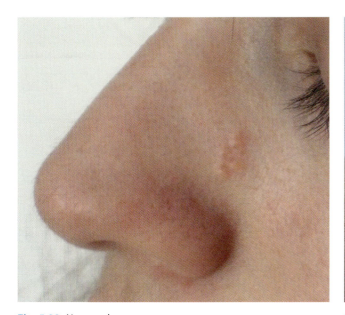

Fig. 5.22. Nevus sebaceus

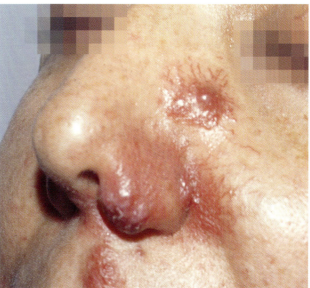

Fig. 5.24. Spider angioma

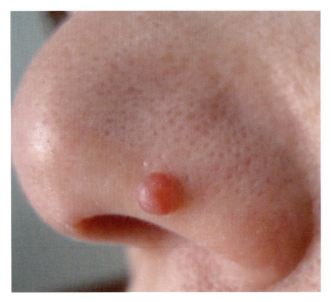

Fig. 5.25. Senile angioma

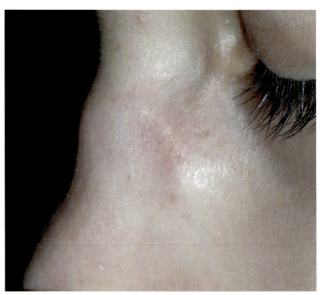

Fig. 5.27. Papular mucinosis

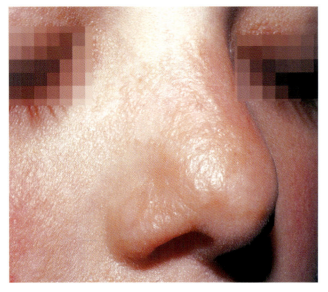

Fig. 5.26. Juvenile colloid milium

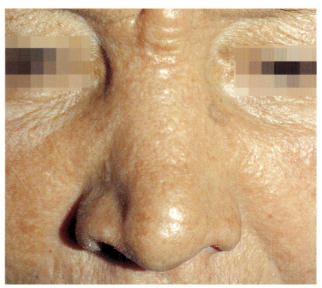

Fig. 5.28. Scleromyxedema

2-4 mm sized facial papules with smooth surface are seen in papular mucinosis and scleromyxedema. These papules caused by mucine storage may be grouped and may form swellings or grooves due to diffuse infiltration on the root of the nose (Figs. 5.27, 5.28). These patients must be investigated in detail for paraproteinemias. In the late phase of erythropoietic protoporphiria waxy papules grouped on the nose, cheeks and also dorsum of the hands can be observed. The skin is thickened with radial fissure-like changes. Besides, atrophic, cribriform scars may occur especially in perioral region of the patients.

Verruca plana is a common HPV infection which presents with flat, smooth-surfaced, flesh- or light brown-coloured papules occurring mostly in puberty and in early adulthood (Fig. 5.29). Like other areas of the face, the nose may frequently be involved. These papules may remain unchanged for a long time. Molluscum contagiosum may sometimes involve the nose (Fig. 5.30). Umbilicated papules on this region can occur due to this *pox virus* infection or cryptococcosis, a deep mycotic infection that is more commonly seen in AIDS patients. Cutaneous cryptococcosis may rarely develop primarily due to direct inoculation by trauma or may develop secondary to hematogenous spread as seen in immunocompromised patients. This infection may also cause meningitis in these patients. The number and morphology of the skin lesions of cryptococcosis differ widely; pustules, nodules, ulcers, subcutaneous abscesses, draining sinuses or cellulitis may occur. Definite diagnosis depends on biopsy and culture. In secondary syphilis, copper-red facial papules with

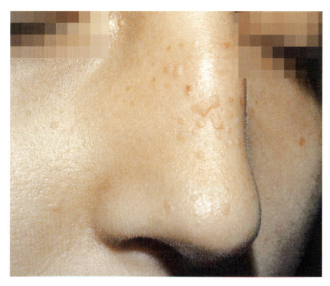

Fig. 5.29. Verruca plana

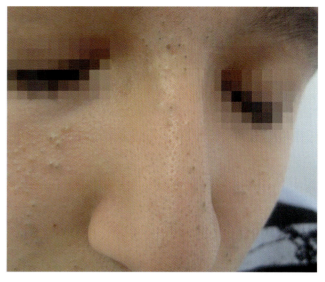

Fig. 5.31. Acne vulgaris. Open comedones

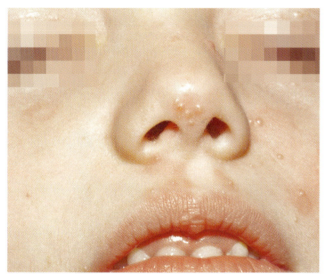

Fig. 5.30. Molluscum contagiosum

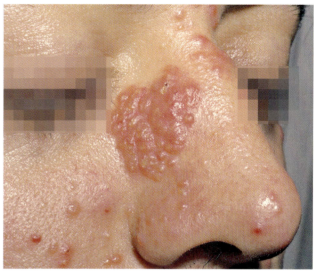

Fig. 5.32. Lupus miliaris disseminatus faciei

thin scales may be observed on the nose and nasolabial folds. Open comedones (blackheads) as tiny, black papules are frequent on the nose in acne vulgaris (Fig. 5.31).

Nasal fold papules occur mostly in children with allergic rhinitis due to the frequent wiping and elevating the nasal tip upwards repeatedly. They resemble linearly arranged milia or comedones on the nose. Epidermodysplasia verruciformis presents with papules clinically resembling verruca plana on the face and vegetating or seborrheic keratosis-like lesions on different parts of the body, appearing in childhood. There is a tendency to the development of squamous cell carcinoma in sun-exposed areas of the body in these patients. Lupus miliaris disseminatus faciei is a chronic granulomatous disease presenting with many small brownish red papules on the eyelids, cheeks, chin, forehead and also on the nose. Papules can rarely be seen as grouped in this form of tuberculids (Fig. 5.32). Lesions may heal leaving atrophic scars. The tiny papular lesions of sarcoidosis may involve the nose as well as other parts of the face.

Trichostasis spinulosa is an idiopathic disease that occurs as a result of the retention of unmedullated vellus hairs in hair follicles and is mostly located on the nose. It presents as deposition of a black material, especially on the follicular openings of the nasal tip and ala nasi where the extending hairs may be noticed easily, and only poses a cosmetic problem. Cyclosporine-induced folliculodystrophy is a rare cutaneous adverse drug reaction. Flesh-coloured, tiny, abundant, follicular papules occur on the nose, midface and ears. Dystrophic hairs or hair-like keratinous spicules may be seen on top of these papules.

6 ■ Nodular Lesions

Substantial part of the nodules located on the nose is due to benign or malignant tumors. Infections, storage disorders and inflammatory diseases may also cause nodules on this area. Additionally, some congenital abnormalities may also be present on the nose with a nodule since their predilection to localize on the midline.

Nasal glioma is a rare benign, congenital midline lesion that occurs as a result of the brain tissue locating outside the cranial closure lines. This type of neural heterotopia mostly presents as a firm, incompressible, pinky or purple, hemangioma-like nodule 1-2 cm in diameter occurring on the nasal bridge or near the nasal root. Some lesions may be connected with the brain. Thus, before performing a biopsy, a neural imaging procedure should be performed. Nasal glioma does not involute spontaneously. Dermoid cyst appears as a congenital flesh-coloured, firm or rubber-like, painless nodule which can be observed anywhere on the midline, from glabella to the nasal tip. Lateral aspects of the face and anterior aspect of the neck are other possible sites for its occurence.

A sinus tract and a tuft of protruding hairs may be observed on the cyst (Fig. 6.1). This special clinical type is called median nasal dermoid fistule. There may be an intracranial connection mostly in cases with sinus tracts. Another congenital midline lesion, encephalocele, occurs as a blue-coloured, soft nodule showing pits when pressed. This neural-tissue containing mass can be pulsatile.

Different types of melanocytic nevi (moles) may involve the nose. Among these, intradermal nevus is frequently observed as approximately 1 cm sized, light brown- or flesh-coloured lesion with a few protruding hairs (Figs. 6.2, 6.3). Especially adult women may have several lesions together. These nevi remain unchanged for years and may only cause a cosmetic problem. Congenital melanocytic nevi can be bigger than the acquired ones, and they may sometimes cover the whole nasal surface (Figs. 6.4, 6.5). These lesions are usually dark-coloured and may be covered with hairs. It is necessary to avoid sun exposure in patients with facial congenital nevi. Spitz nevus presents with brown or pink, smooth-surfaced,

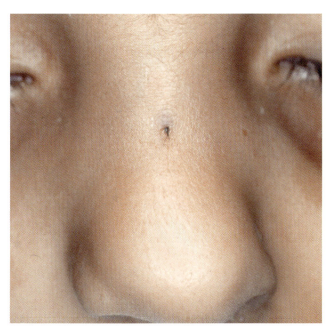

Fig. 6.1. Median nasal dermoid fistule

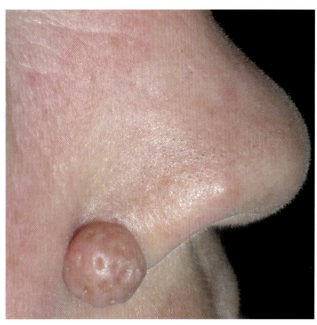

Fig. 6.2. Intradermal melanocytic nevus

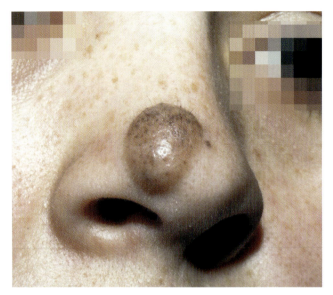

Fig. 6.3. Intradermal melanocytic nevus

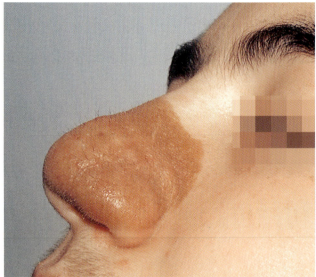

Fig. 6.5. Congenital melanocytic nevus

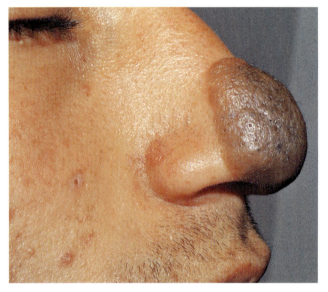

Fig. 6.4. Congenital melanocytic nevus

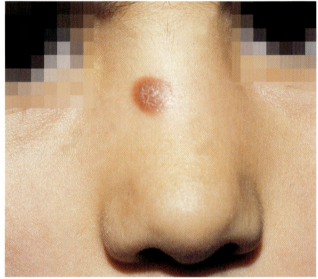

Fig. 6.6. Spitz nevus

dome-shaped, approximately 1 cm sized solitary nodules on the nose and on the other areas of the face as well (Fig. 6.6). Most commonly, it appears during childhood and remains unchanged. As its histopathological features resemble malignant melanoma, it is also called "juvenile melanoma". However, the risk for malignant transformation is very low in Spitz nevus. Though not common, blue nevus may be seen as grey, bluish or black papules or nodules on the nose (Fig. 6.7).

Lentigo malignant melanoma, a tumor which has a well-known relationship with cumulative effects of ultraviolet light, should be considered especially in elderly patients with nasal patches or plaques with indistinct borders and irregular pigmentation (Fig. 6.8). Signs of invasive stage are brown or black papules and nodules which develop on the neglected plaques. The surface of these nodules may be intact or ulcerated. At this stage, the prognosis is substantially worse. Nodal and visceral metastases may also occur at this stage. Desmoplastic malignant melanoma is a rare type of malignant melanoma that may sometimes appear on the nose as a pigmented or flesh-coloured, indurated, fibrotic tissue-like nodule or plaque. Although metastases are rare in this type, tumor may invade deep tissues, and recurrences may be seen frequently after inadequate excision. On the other hand, malignant melanoma may occasionally arise from nasal mucosa or paranasal sinuses (sinonasal mucosal melanoma). The mucosal lesion may present as a sessile mass and lead to unilateral nasal obstruction or nasal bleeding. In advanced stages, invasion of adjacent tissues and metastases may occur.

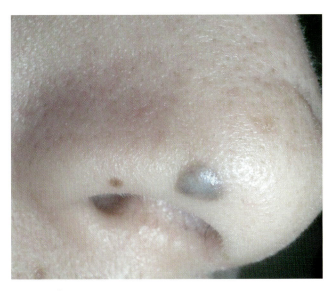

Fig. 6.7. Blue nevus

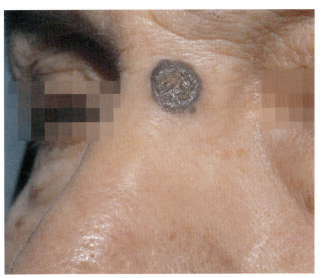

Fig. 6.9. Basal cell carcinoma. Pigmented type

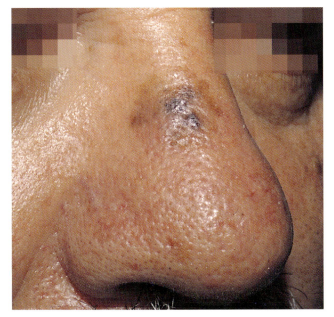

Fig. 6.8. Lentigo malignant melanoma

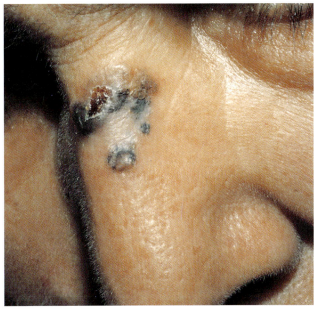

Fig. 6.10. Basal cell carcinoma. Pigmented type

A frequent cause of nasal nodules is basal cell carcinoma which mostly occurs as a flesh- or pink-coloured but sometimes hyperpigmented lesion (Figs. 6.9, 6.10). Its superficial type appears rarely on the nose as a flat plaque (Fig. 6.11). Nodulo-ulcerative and cystic types of this tumor starts as a papule and reach 1-2 cm size over a long period of time (Figs. 6.12, 6.13). Morpheaform type of basal cell carcinoma is observed as firm, fibrotic plaques (Fig. 6.14). Untreated tumors may invade deep tissues, in extremely rare cases metastasize. Tumors located on the upper part of the nose mostly infiltrate the periosteum whereas tumors on the lower parts infiltrate the perichondrium. In large, long-standing tumors, more aggressive treatments should be given which can lead to unpleasant cosmetic results (Fig. 6.15). Thus, early diagnosis of basal cell carcinoma is crucial. Both the nasolabial sulcus and the nose per se are high risk areas for recurrence. A type of in situ carcinoma, Bowen's disease, may arise as a slowly-growing, slightly raised solitary plaque, with a well-demarcated border. When treated early, the risk of transforming to squamous cell carcinoma is low.

The nose is a well-known location for lymphocytoma cutis, the most frequently seen type of pseudolymphomas. Though various antigenic stimuli triggering lymphocytoma cutis have been described, in most cases the cause cannot be identified.

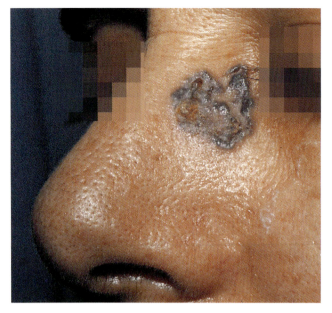

Fig. 6.11. Basal cell carcinoma. Superficial-pigmented type

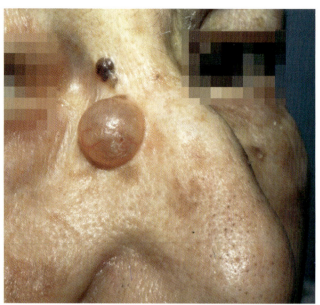

Fig. 6.13. Basal cell carcinoma. Cystic type

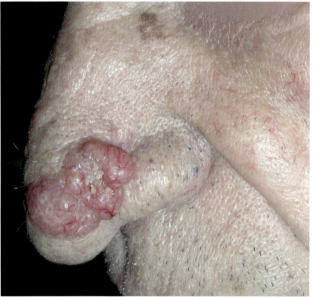

Fig. 6.12. Basal cell carcinoma. Nodulo-ulcerative type

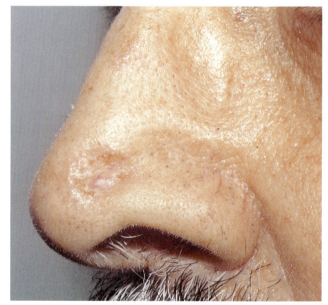

Fig. 6.14. Basal cell carcinoma. Morpheaform type

Smooth, asymptomatic, erythematous, plum-coloured papules or nodules arise mostly on ala nasi and nasal tip. They remain unchanged after reaching a certain size on average of 1-1.5 cm (Figs. 6.16-6.18). Although the disease resembles lymphomas in terms of histopathologic characteristics, it is benign and does not lead to visceral involvement. Pseudolymphomas may be treated with intralesional injection of corticosteroids. Distinguishing these lesions from marginal zone lymphoma (Figs. 6.19, 6.20), a low-grade cutaneous B cell lymphoma which rarely arises on the nose, is only possible by immunohistochemical methods and molecular biological examinations used to determine monoclonality. Small-medium pleomorphic T cell lymphoma may also appear on the face and sometimes on the nose as a solitary erythematous or purplish nodule.

Unlike patch or plaque lesions, tumoral lesions occurring during the tumor-stage of mycosis fungoides may often involve sun-exposed areas such as the face (Fig. 6.21). Reddish tumors on the nose may reach a large size sometimes in a very short time. After the tumoral lesions become evident, the prognosis of this cutaneous T cell lymphoma worsens. Papules and nodules seen in lymphomatoid papulosis may

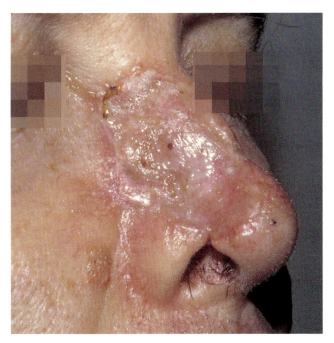

Fig. 6.15. Basal cell carcinoma. After surgery

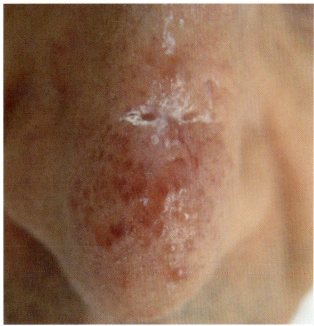

Fig. 6.17. Pseudolymphoma. Lymphocytoma cutis

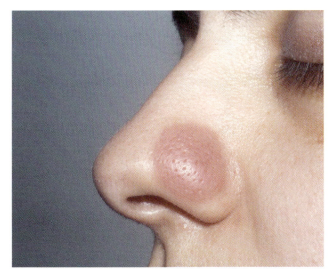

Fig. 6.16. Pseudolymphoma. Lymphocytoma cutis

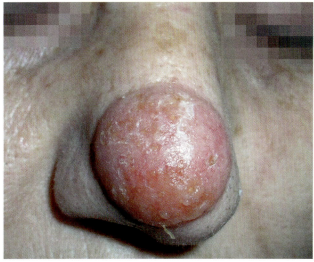

Fig. 6.18. Pseudolymphoma. Lymphocytoma cutis

sometimes be located on the nose (Fig. 6.22). The lesions of this low-grade cutaneous T cell lymphoma are self limiting but recurrent. Cutaneous leukemia rarely leads to diffuse induration of the nasal skin.

The nose and the nasolabial sulcus are among the common sites of involvement with microcystic adnexal carcinoma, an adnexal tumor of the skin showing apocrine differentiation. Slowly-growing, pale yellow, firm nodules and plaques have indistinct borders and may involve deep tissues. This tumor has a high recurrence rate but usually does not metastasize. Sebaceous carcinoma, a tumor showing sebaceous gland differentiation, may occasionally be located on the nose as a yellow or pinkish nodule with telangiectatic vessels especially in elderly patients. Their presence should be considered as a marker for Muir-Torre syndrome. Merkel cell carcinoma, an aggressive neuroendocrine tumor, preferentially appears on sun-exposed areas such as the face, neck and scalp, and may lead to firm, nontender, violaceous or purple nodular lesions on the nose. It has a potential for regional and distant metastases. Olfactory neuroblastoma originates from cranial nerve I which terminates on the nose and may cause nodules on this region. Presenting initially with epistaxis and anosmia, this tumor may grow to large masses in advanced stages.

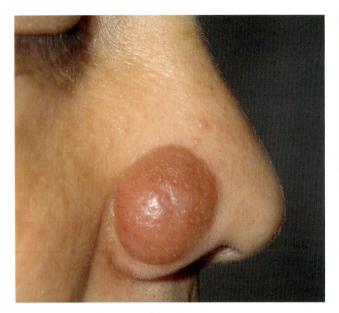

Fig. 6.19. Marginal zone B cell lymphoma

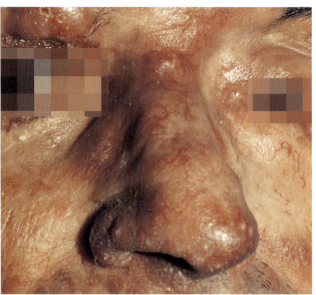

Fig. 6.21. Mycosis fungoides

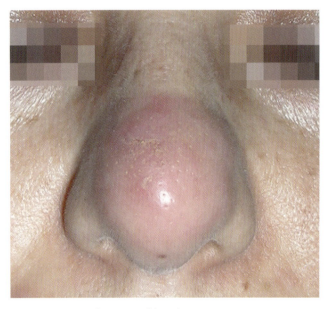

Fig. 6.20. Marginal zone B cell lymphoma

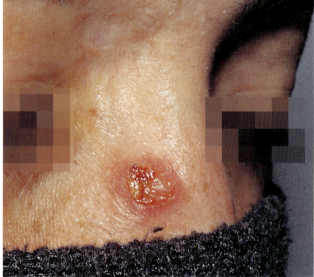

Fig. 6.22. Lymphomatoid papulosis

Cutaneous metastases resulting from solid malignancies occasionally involve the nose, and may emerge suddenly as firm nodules and infiltrated plaques. Although rare, lung cancer, breast cancer, renal cell carcinoma and chordoma are among the tumors which are known to metastasize to the nose. Following the skin metastases, the prognosis of internal organ tumors worsens. Keratoacanthoma frequently locates on the nose as a rapidly-growing, solitary, exophytic, 1-2 cm sized nodule with a central horny plug and punched out border (Fig. 6.23). The tumor is adherent to the underlying tissue. The lesion may heal spontaneously with scarring in a few months to years. However, excision may be required since the clinical appearance does not always allow a clear distinction from the squamous cell carcinoma. Warty dyskeratoma occurs as a solitary flesh- or reddish brown-coloured papule or nodule, ranging from several mm to 2 cm in diameter with a central keratin plug. It may locate on the nose and other parts of the face. It is important in the differential diagnosis of the diseases showing acantholytic dyskeratosis histologically.

Rhinosporidiosis, rhinoscleroma, chronic mucocutaneous candidiasis, actinomycosis, aspergillosis, histoplasmosis, sporotrichosis and blastomycosis are also among the infectious diseases that can occur on the nose and cause infiltrative or

6 Nodular Lesions 43

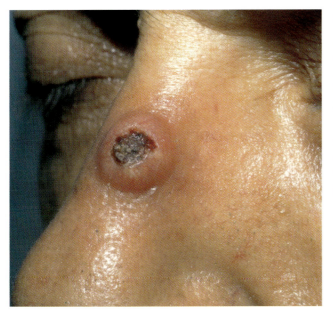
Fig. 6.23. Keratoacanthoma

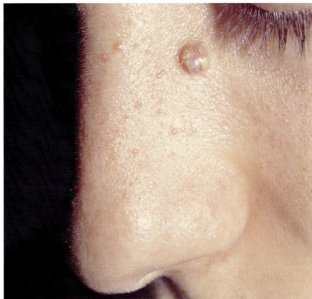
Fig. 6.25. Pilomatricoma

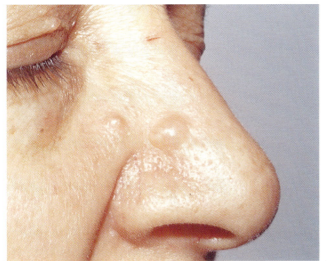
Fig. 6.24. Cylindroma

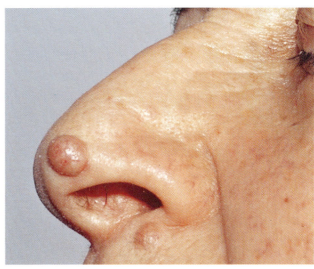
Fig. 6.26. Neurofibromatosis

nodular lesions. Most of them show granulomatous histopathological features and have been mentioned in the related chapter.

Some benign tumors and cysts are observed around the nasal area with nodular lesions. Cylindroma is a tumor of sweat gland epithelium characterized by slowly-growing, pink, red or bluish nodule that has a rubber-like consistency (Fig. 6.24). Familial cases may occur with multiple lesions and these acquired tumors may reach several centimeters in size. Although it is accepted as a benign tumor, it rarely shows malignant transformation. A tumor with epithelial and mesenchymal differentiation, chondroid syringoma (mixed tumor of skin), occurs during adulthood and causes flesh-coloured, 0.5 to 3 cm intradermal and subcutaneous nodules on the nose.

Pilomatricoma (calcifying epithelioma of Malherbe), a hamartoma of the hair follicle matrix, may be seen on the nose as a firm solitary nodule with anetodermic surface in different colours (Fig. 6.25). There may be many neurofibromas in patients with neurofibromatosis (Figs. 6.26, 6.27). A helpful diagnostic clue is the invagination of neurofibroma when applied pressure with the fingertip. Epidermoid cyst is a mobile nodule with a smooth surface and central punctum

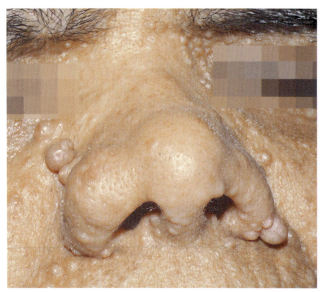

Fig. 6.27. Neurofibromatosis

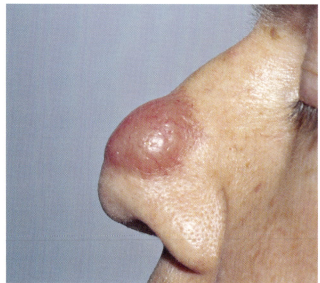

Fig. 6.29. Epidermoid cyst

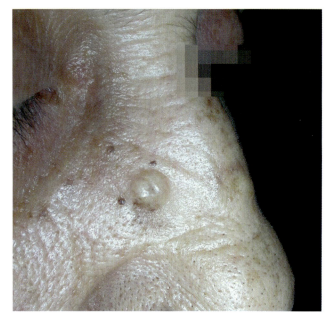

Fig. 6.28. Epidermoid cyst

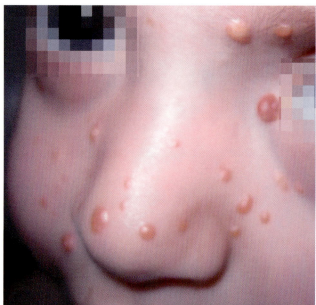

Fig. 6.30. Juvenile xanthogranuloma

and may range from several mm to cm in size (Figs. 6.28, 6.29). When compressed, a cheese-like material can be protruded from the center. Cystic lesions of basal cell carcinoma may also be misdiagnosed as the benign tumors mentioned above (Fig. 6.13).

Juvenile xanthogranuloma is the most common type of non-Langerhans cell histiocytoses. It is characterized by yellowish to orange-coloured, asymptomatic papules or nodules most frequently seen in infants and children (Fig. 6.30). Lesions may be located on many parts of the body as well as on the nose. The size of these lesions vary. In addition to the typical round or oval solitary nodules of 1-2 cm in diameter, numerous 2-5 mm sized, firm, hemispheric papules may also be seen. Even the multiple lesions do not show tendency to cluster. Most patients are otherwise healthy. However, the eye, lung, bone and central nervous system may occasionally be affected. Surgical interventions should be avoided for the self-limiting cutaneous lesions that improve within 3-6 years with little scarring (Fig. 6.31), since these procedures can cause undesirable cosmetic results.

Many types of vascular tumors can be observed on the nose. Infantile capillary hemangiomas are generally seen in 1-3% of the newborns as solitary or several, soft, red

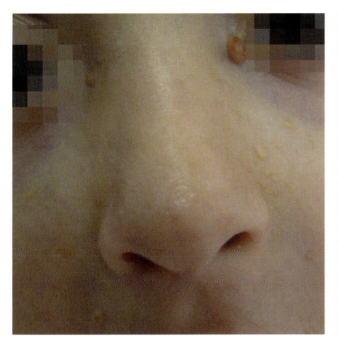

Fig. 6.31. Juvenile xanthogranuloma. Regressing lesion

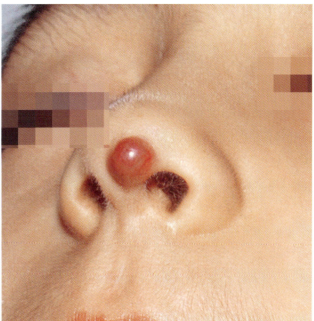

Fig. 6.33. Infantile capillary hemangioma

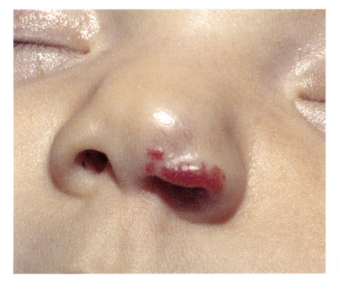

Fig. 6.32. Infantile capillary hemangioma

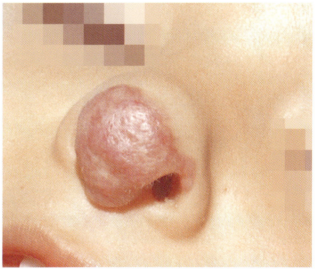

Fig. 6.34. Infantile capillary hemangioma. Cyrano nose

nodules or plaques that vary in size. Together with the other parts of the face, the nose is an important site for these hemangiomas (Figs. 6.32, 6.33). Two distinct forms with different courses can be distinguished; superficial and deep types according to the level of benign vascular proliferation in the dermis. Deep hemangiomas of the nasal tip may cause a special appearance of the nose with a bulbous prominence which is called as the "Cyrano" or "Pinocchio" nose (Fig. 6.34). These hemangiomas may ulcerate and invade the cartilage which results in the development of fibrous tissue. For large hemangiomas that obstruct nostrils and cause respiratory difficulty, intralesional or systemic highdose corticosteroid may be administered to reduce the tumor size. On the other hand small and superficial infantile capillary hemangiomas tend to regress spontaneously before 7 years of age. It should be kept in mind that large, unilateral plaque-like facial hemangiomas (Fig. 6.35) may be part of PHACES syndrome. Therefore, appropriate investigations should be performed to search for the presence of cerebral artery abnormalities, posterior fossa malformations, aort coarctation and ipsilateral microphtalmy.

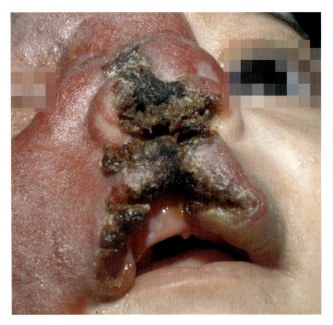

Fig. 6.35. Infantile capillary hemangioma

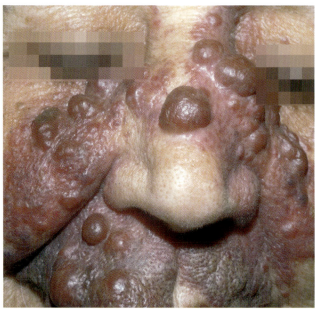

Fig. 6.37. Nevus flammeus. Late stage

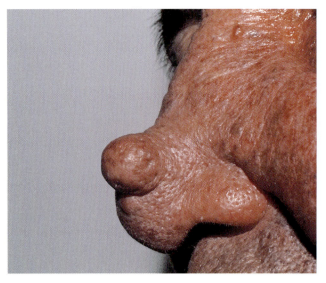

Fig. 6.36. Nevus flammeus. Late stage

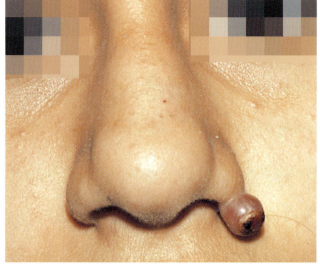

Fig. 6.38. Pyogenic granuloma

Lymphangioma, schwannoma, cutaneous metastasis, Kaposi's sarcoma and juvenile xanthogranuloma are other lesions which may cause the "Cyrano nose" when they are located on the nasal tip. Red or purple puffy nodules may develop on the port-wine-stain type of nevus flammeus which is a congenital, flat lesion (Figs. 6.36, 6.37). Pyogenic granuloma is a type of hemangioma which occur at any age group as a red, dome-shaped or stalky, friable, 0.5-1 cm sized nodule with an eroded surface on the nose, around nostrils and at the border of mucosa (Figs. 6.38, 6.39). An epidermal collarette supports the diagnosis. It is commonly observed in pregnancy. Spindle cell hemangioendothelioma is mostly observed on distal extremities as a slowly-growing, red brown-coloured papule or nodule, but may also occur on the nose. This tumor has a tendency to recur and is usually seen in Maffucci or Klippel-Trenaunay-Weber syndromes. It has been speculated that this lesion develops due to an alteration in local blood flow. Therefore, it may regress when the underlying vascular event resolves. Hobnail hemangioma which shows a typical cell morphology mostly arises on the extremities and trunk, but may also be located on the nose.

Among the facial lesions of Kaposi's sarcoma, nasal location has a special importance. Apart from early macular lesions, it generally occurs as purple-coloured nodules which may sometimes be ulcerated (Fig. 6.40). The tumor occasionally arises from nasal mucosa. Bacillary angiomatosis

6 Nodular Lesions

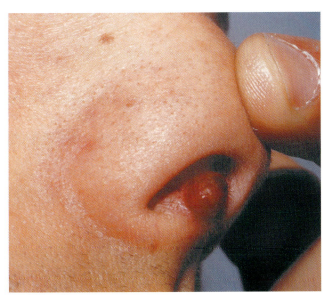

Fig. 6.39. Pyogenic granuloma

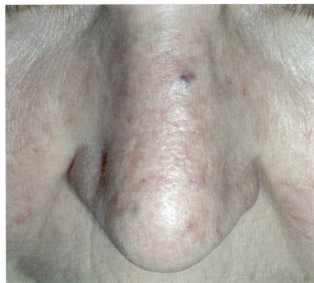

Fig. 6.41. Venous lake

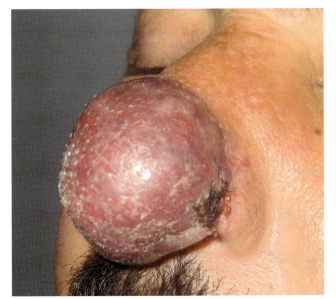

Fig. 6.40. Kaposi's sarcoma. Cyrano nose

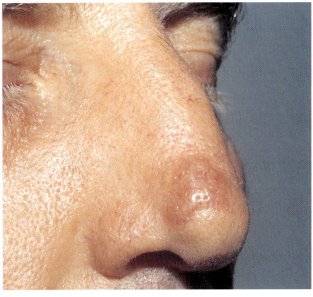

Fig. 6.42. Granuloma faciale

is a bartonella infection, which mostly occurs in AIDS or post transplant patients. Rapidly-growing, reddish purple, round, pyogenic granuloma-like papules and nodules may be observed on the face and nose. Ulceration and bleeding may also occur. The dramatic response to antibiotic treatment confirms the diagnosis and prevents dissemination. In Bonnet- Dechaume-Blanc syndrome, the skin is initially red, slightly infiltrated and warm due to arteriovenous malformation mainly in the midline of the face including the nose. Infiltration increases over time, and auscultation reveals a thrill-like sound. Complications such as necrosis and ulceration may develop. In the late stages of this arterio-venous malformation, as well as epistaxis and nasal congestion, there may also be other symptoms due to eye (retina) and brain involvement. Venous lake is an idiopathic acquired angiomatous lesion which rarely leads to dark blue papules or nodules on the nose (Fig. 6.41).

Granuloma faciale is an idiopathic eosinophilic dermatosis which is mostly located on the nose accompanying a few facial nodular lesions (Figs. 6.42-6.44). An association with systemic diseases has not been established. Most patients are adults over middle age. Follicular openings are visible on the surface of reddish brown or violaceous asymptomatic nodules and plaques. Lesions grow slowly and do

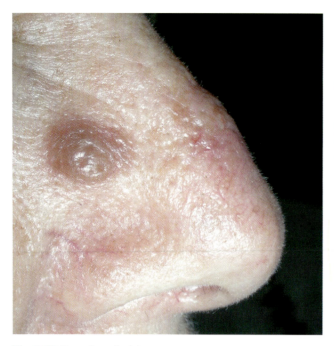

Fig. 6.43. Granuloma faciale

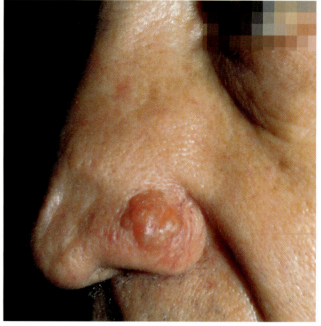

Fig. 6.45. Nodular amyloidosis

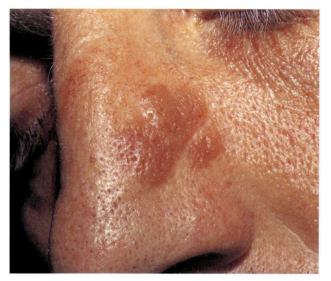

Fig. 6.44. Granuloma faciale

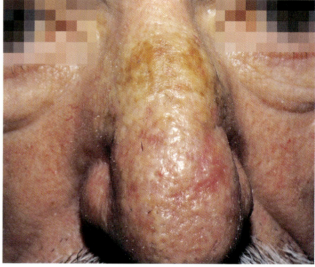

Fig. 6.46. Solar elastosis

not show ulceration. They only cause a cosmetic problem and show no tendency for spontaneous resolution. Even if the lesions are surgically excised, new lesions may occur. The rarest type of primary skin amyloidoses, the nodular amyloidosis, has a predilection to locate on acral regions and also on the nose. Yellowish-brown or pink-coloured, solitary or a few nodules may show telangiectasia and hemorrhagic foci on the surface. Typically, lesions recur at the same location after excision or destruction when they are misdiagnosed as tumors (Fig. 6.45). Yellowish pink papulonodular lesions and plaques of primary systemic amyloidosis may also be seen on the nose. Tendency towards purpura especially on the eyelids, carpal tunnel syndrome, macroglossia, and involvement of multiple internal organs are other features of the disease. These patients should be investigated for multiple myeloma and plasma cell dyscrasia. The nodules may increase in number and become larger even under therapy.

Individuals with fair skin are prone to developing solar elastosis on the nose which appears as yellowish thickened skin areas (Fig. 6.46). Favre-Racouchot syndrome (nodular elastoidosis) is a severe form of chronic ultraviolet light

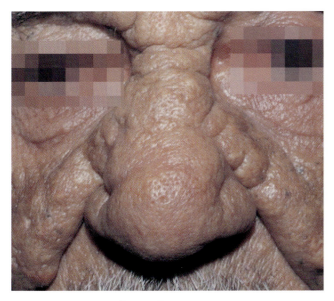

Fig. 6.47. Favre-Racouchot syndrome

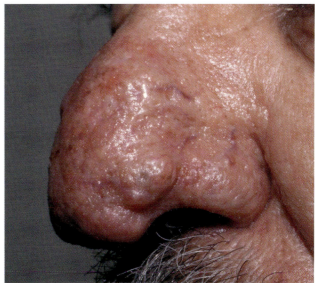

Fig. 6.49. Phymatous rosacea

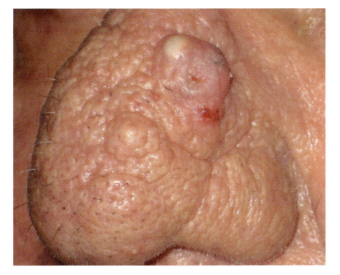

Fig. 6.48. Phymatous rosacea

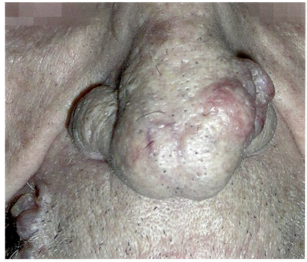

Fig. 6.50. Phymatous rosacea

damage and presents with yellowish elastoid nodules. These lesions commonly occur on the nose as well as on the cheeks (Fig. 6.47). The disease is typically observed in elderly men. Other features of dermatoheliosis like senile comedones may accompany the nodules.

Phymatous rosacea is a sebaceous gland hyperplasia particularly accompanying severe rosacea in elderly men. However, a history of rosacea is not present in every patient. Lesions mostly occur on the nose where the sebaceous glands are dense (rhinophyma). Pilosebaceous poral orifices are prominent in the affected area (Fig. 6.48). The severity of erythema is variable, the skin may be reddish or purple in colour, and there may be overlying telangiectases (Fig. 6.49). It usually involves the lower two thirds of the nose; and is prominent on the tip and ala nasi. The skin of the nose is thickened with irregular nodules and lobules (Fig. 6.50). Sometimes, there may be pendulous masses which cause severe cosmetic problem. In severe cases nasal breathing may be impaired. Basal cell carcinoma may occasionally develop on rhinophyma. Electrosurgery and carbondioxide laser may be used especially in severe cases to remove the excessive and hyperplastic tissues. On the other hand, it should be kept in mind that nose lesions of granuloma faciale, hemangiomas, basal cell carcinoma, angiosarcoma, cutaneous lymphomas, cutaneous metastases, cylindroma, tuberous sclerosis and cryptococcosis may sometimes mimick rhinophyma.

Orf is a *pox virus* infection, which spreads mostly as a result of direct contact with sheep or goats. It may occasionally

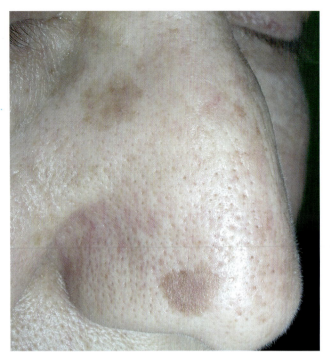

Fig. 6.51. Seborrheic keratosis

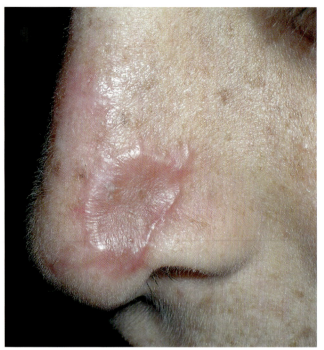

Fig. 6.53. Hypertropic scar (on the site of excision)

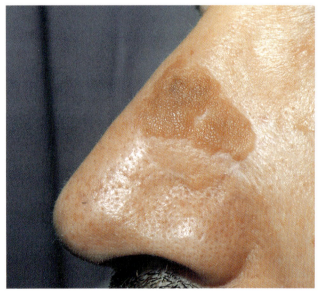

Fig. 6.52. Seborrheic keratosis

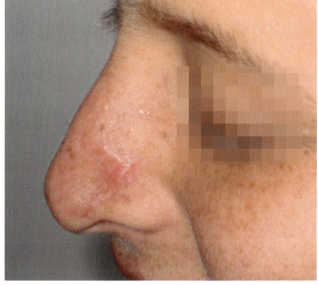

Fig. 6.54. Hypertropic scar (regressing lesion)

be located on other body areas apart from the typical location on the hands. When target-like solitary nodules appear on the nose, one should also consider orf. In some patients, there may be several lesions. During the course of the disease, a papillomatous appearance may occur on the surface of the nodule. A history of recent contact with animals supports the diagnosis. The lesions heal in about 4-6 weeks without scarring.

However, misdiagnosis may lead to unnecessary surgical interventions resulting with unwanted scars.

One of the most common benign tumors of the skin, seborrheic keratosis, may present with dirty yellow-, brown- or black-coloured, well-demarcated, verrucous or papillomatous nodules on the nose (Figs. 6.51, 6.52). Lesions are approximately 8-10 mm in diameter and do not lead to subjective complaints. However, irritation of tumors may cause erythema and itching. Most patients are over the middle age and have other lesions on different parts of the body. These tumors are treated only for cosmetic reasons. Nevus lipomatosis superficialis is a hamartomatous lesion mostly seen on the hip and lumbosacral region, but it may occasionally be located on the nose as flesh-coloured, soft papules and nodules.

In Costello syndrome which is considered as a variant of Noonan syndrome, papillomas emerge around the nose and mouth. Thick and loose skin appearance on the dorsal areas of hands and feet accompanied by deep palmoplantar creases are the main features of the disease. Furthermore, calcified epitheliomas, dermoid cysts, syringomas and fibroadenomas of the breast may also be seen in this disease.

Although the nose is not a common area for keloid formation, it should be remembered that a hypertrophic scar may develop here following surgical interventions (Fig. 6.53). Unlike keloid, hypertrophic scars improve spontaneously in about one year (Fig. 6.54).

7 ■ Granulomatous Lesions

Plaques may be observed alongside papules and nodules in diseases with granulomatous histopathology. In this chapter, primarily granulomatous diseases presenting with nodules and plaques will be mentioned. Diseases mostly presenting with papules with granulomatous histopathology were discussed in the "papular lesions" chapter. As granulomatous nodules can definitely be differentiated from other nodules with different etiologies only by histopathological means, diseases mentioned here may clinically be confused with the ones in the "nodular lesions" chapter. Although the granulomatous diseases mainly affect the nasal skin initially, they may also involve the nasal mucosa in the chronic stage and be destructive. Most of the granulomatous conditions affecting the nose are specific chronic infections or infestations, but some are inflammatory dermatoses which cause granulomatous lesions on this area.

Cutaneous leishmaniasis can present with a granulomatous plaque of coalescing papules, especially in the late phase or in relapse (chronic lupoid leishmaniasis) (Figs. 7.1, 7.2). In lepromatous leprosy, there may be erythematous nodules and plaques on the nose. The skin of the nose appears to be thickened due to diffuse infiltration (Figs. 7.3, 7.4). Granulomatous plaques may also exist in other parts of the body. Loss of eyebrows may be a sign of facial involvement. Diffuse infiltration and nodules can also be observed on the nasal mucosa. Chronic nasal obstruction, epistaxis and formation of crust are typical signs of intranasal involvement. In later stages of the disease, underlying cartilage and bone may be destroyed leading to nasal septum deviation and "saddle nose" deformity. Nasal secretion contains numerous bacteria (*Mycobacterium leprae*) in untreated patients. Therefore smear samples can be obtained from the nasal mucosa for the diagnosis of leprosy.

Lupus vulgaris, the most common form of skin tuberculosis, favors especially the nose, ears or cheeks in the head and neck region (Figs. 7.5-7.8). Hematogenous transmission

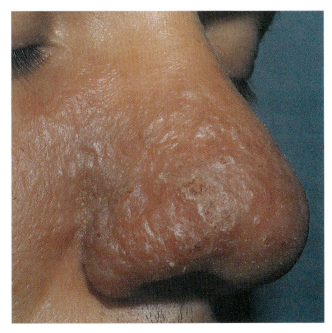

Fig. 7.1. Cutaneous leishmaniasis

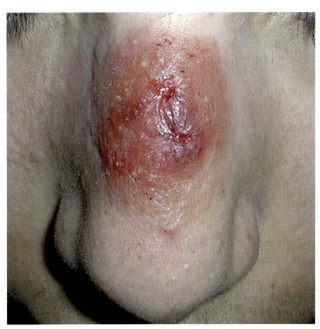

Fig. 7.2. Cutaneous leishmaniasis

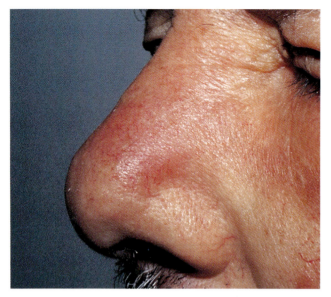

Fig. 7.3. Leprosy

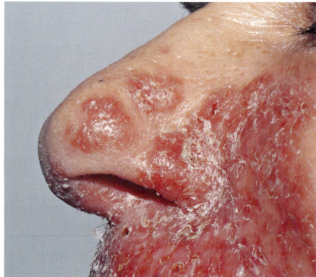

Fig. 7.5. Lupus vulgaris

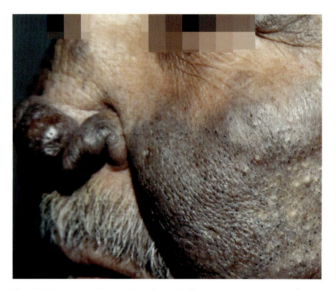

Fig. 7.4. Leprosy (the patient has also hyperpigmentation induced by clofazimine)

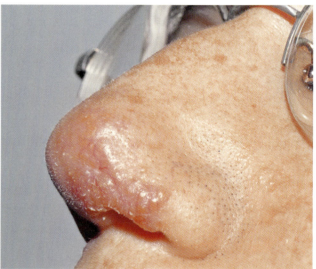

Fig. 7.6. Lupus vulgaris

is implicated for the nasal lesions. Adults are more commonly affected. The initial lesions are usually small papules that slowly enlarge and coalesce to form a plaque. A well-demarcated single plaque is soft and red-brown usually with smooth surface. However, hyperkeratosis or scales may sometimes be seen on the plaques. "Apple-jelly" colour can be seen when pressed with a glass slide (diascopy). Granulomas with central caseation necrosis is typical histopathological feature of lupus vulgaris but may not be present in all cases. The causative organism (*Mycobacterium tuberculosis*) is also hard to be seen microscopically. The tuberculine test is highly positive. Active internal tuberculosis may only be rarely detected in patients with lupus vulgaris. As the lesions are typically asymptomatic, some patients consult physicians in the late stage. In such cases, the destruction of the nasal cartilage may be a complication of the disease. Standard antituberculosis therapy is indicated for cutaneous tuberculosis.

The tertiary (late) stage of syphilis, a sexually transmitted infection caused by *Treponema pallidum,* is rarely seen today. It may present with granulomatous nodules and plaques on the nose resembling lupus vulgaris in early untreated cases. Serologic testing must be performed to confirm the diagnosis. Rhinoscleroma is a chronic progressive infectious

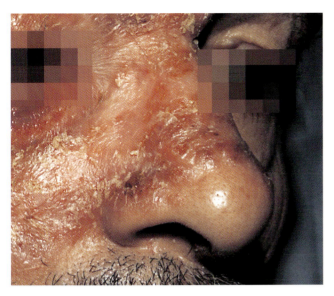

Fig. 7.7. Lupus vulgaris

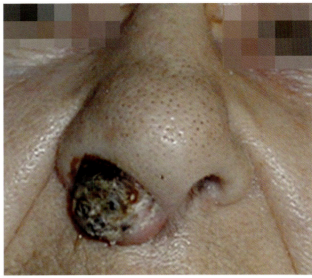

Fig. 7.9. Rhinosporidiosis

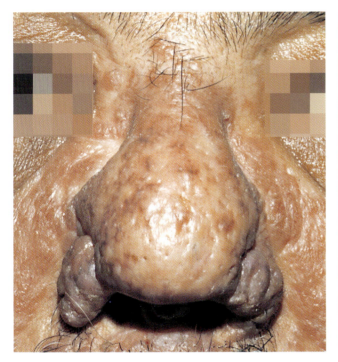

Fig. 7.8. Lupus vulgaris

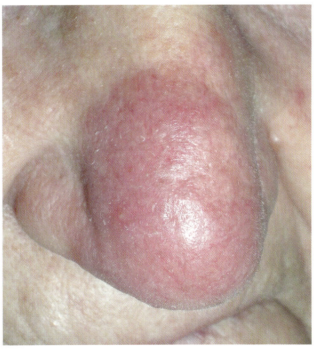

Fig. 7.10. Sarcoidosis. Lupus pernio

disease which affects the nose, pharynx and the adjacent structures. The causative agent is *Klebsiella pneumoniae spp. rhinoscleromatis*. It begins with a chronic rhinitis and crusting which is resistant to medical therapies. Then, reddish brown, firm nodules or sclerotic plaques showing granulomatous infiltration histopathologically gradually develop around the nasal vestibule. In the advanced stages obstruction of the nares may occur. Some of the deep (systemic) mycosis can also cause granulomatous lesions on the nose. Rhinosporidiosis, a deep mycosis caused by *Rhinosporidium seeberi*, may arise as pedunculated nodules on the nasal mucosa (Fig. 7.9). Pink-, red- or purple-coloured, soft polypoid lesions, especially when located close to the nostrils, may cover, and even obstruct the vestibule. Treatment of choice is excision since antifungal and antimicrobial drugs do not show significant efficacy.

Cutananeous sarcoidosis occurs in up to one third of patients with systemic sarcoidosis. Lupus pernio is the most characteristic cutaneous lesion of this multisystemic disease with typical granulomatous histopathology (naked tubercles) and especially favors the nose. Violaceous with a cyanosis-like hue or blue-brown, soft plaques with a smooth-surface are seen on the nose symmetrically (Figs. 7.10-7.14). The skin around the nares may seem swollen due to infiltration. The persistent plaques may also spread to adjacent areas of the face. Nasal mucosa may also be involved in some cases in the form of yellowish subcutaneous nodules and polypoid tissue formation. It is particularly disfiguring, and if left untreated, complications such as nasal obstruction, ulceration and collapse of the nasal bridge can be seen. Chronic fibrotic respiratory tract involvement and lytic bone lesions usually accompany lupus pernio. The cutaneous lesions of this chronic disease respond well to systemic corticosteroids, but recurrences may occur.

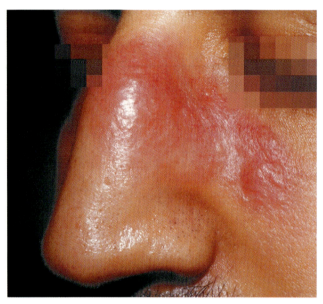

Fig. 7.11. Sarcoidosis. Lupus pernio

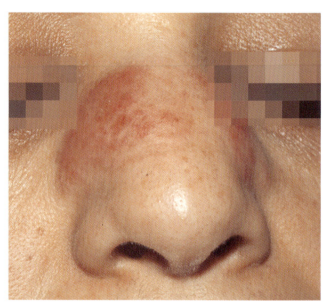

Fig. 7.13. Sarcoidosis. Lupus pernio

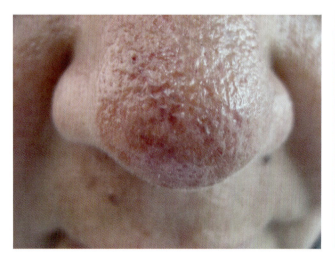

Fig. 7.12. Sarcoidosis. Lupus pernio

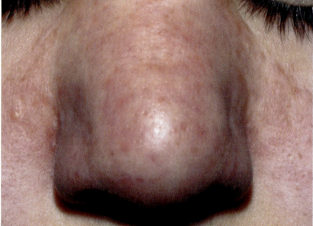

Fig. 7.14. Sarcoidosis. Lupus pernio

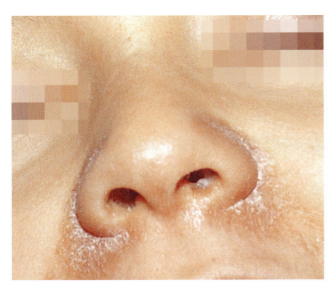
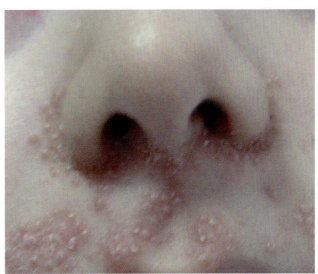

Fig. 7.15. Granulomatous periorifical dermatitis

Fig. 7.16. Granulomatous periorificial dermatitis

Acanthoma fissuratum develops mostly behind the ears due to the mechanical trauma of ill-fitting glasses, but may sometimes be seen on the lateral aspects of the nasal bridge as flesh-coloured or erythematous nodules and plaques. These granulomatous lesion is often clinically mistaken for a basal cell carcinoma on the nose. The diagnosis is confirmed by histopathological examination together with the history of trauma. Thus, the use of needless therapeutic procedures can be avoided. Granulomatous periorifical dermatitis is a rare idiopathic granulomatous disease which is limited to perioral, perinasal and periocular parts of the face and occurs typically in prepubertal children. It is characterized with yellowish-brown papules which coalesce to form plaques. Nasolabial folds and ala nasi can be involved symmetrically (Figs. 7.15, 7.16). The condition is not associated with systemic involvement. Spontaneous healing frequently occurs after a long period without scarring or post-inflammatory pigmentation.

8 ■ Deformities

Permanent structural deviation of the nose resulting in major shape and size changes (deformity) can be attributed to different etiological factors. The nose may become smaller or larger, thinned or broadened and depressed or sharpened due to various reasons. Cartilage plays an important role in the shape of the nose. Destruction of the cartilage by chronic infections, granulomatous diseases, vasculitis and malignancies are main causes of nasal deformity. Increase in dermal connective tissue in sclerotic diseases, loss of subcutaneous tissue in panniculitis and recurrent blistering diseases resulting with scars may also change the shape of the nose. Deformities can be congenital as observed in some genodermatoses with prominent facial dysmorphism. Therefore, the nose is an important site of evaluation for dysmorphism. In this chapter, the above-mentioned issues will be discussed. Nasal deformities related to genetic diseases without other dermatological signs and enlargement of the nose due to nodular lesions are outside the scope of this chapter. At the end of the chapter nasal lines and grooves will be mentioned briefly.

Lupus vulgaris may cause destruction of the nasal cartilage if not treated appropriately, especially in patients who are immunosuppressed (Fig. 8.1). Tissue loss due to granulomatous infiltration generally starts from the nasal tip. The nose may become beak-like or sometimes a substantial part of the nose, including cartilage, may be destructed in this type of cutaneous tuberculosis (Fig. 8.2). On the other hand, the nasal bone is mostly protected. A recently described syndrome with low surface expression of HLA class I molecules is characterized by chronic necrotizing granulomatous lesions in the upper respiratory tract and skin in addition to cutaneous vasculitis, recurrent respiratory tract infections and

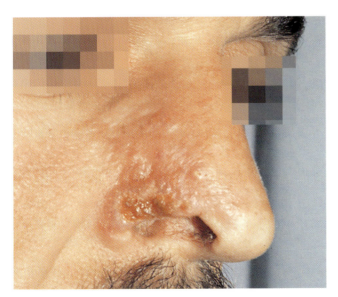

Fig. 8.1. Lupus vulgaris

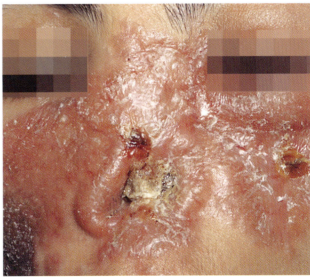

Fig. 8.2. Lupus vulgaris (in an immunosuppressed patient)

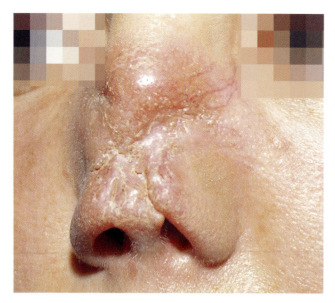

Fig. 8.3. Granulomatous lesions in a patient with low surface expression of HLA class I molecules

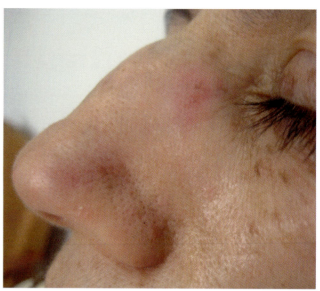

Fig. 8.5. Lupus panniculitis

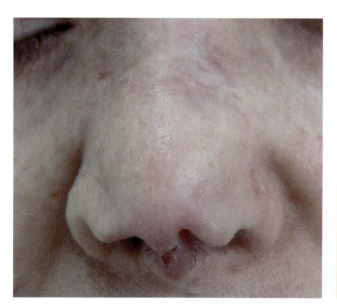

Fig. 8.4. Nasal deformity in a patient with low surface expression of HLA class I molecules

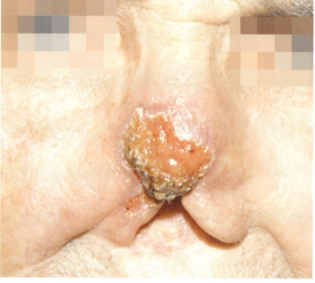

Fig. 8.6. Basal cell carcinoma. Radiotherapy damage

bronchiectasia. Granulomatous plaques may cause severe nasal destruction in these patients (Figs. 8.3, 8.4). The subcutaneous form of lupus erythematosus, lupus panniculitis (lupus profundus), may occasionally be located on the nose. Atrophy of the subcutaneous tissue (lipoatrophy) may cause a smaller nose which may be regionally depressed in the late stage (Fig. 8.5). A substantial number of patients also have erythematous plaques of discoid lupus erythematosus overlying the panniculitis or in other areas.

Both basal cell and squamous cell carcinomas affect the nose frequently. Both tumors can be cured by surgical methods or radiotherapy when diagnosed early. When not treated, unpleasant destruction of the nose may occur due to the invasion of cartilage and bone. High dose radiotherapy given for malignancies may also damage the nasal septum (Fig. 8.6), and cause sinking of the nose. In Gorlin syndrome (Fig. 8.7) and xeroderma pigmentosum (Fig. 8.8) there may be a mild regional collapse on the nose resulting from surgical excision or grafting of recurrent basal cell carcinomas. Odontogenic keratocysts, skeletal abnormalities, hypertelorism, frontal bossing and eye involvement are other manifestations of Gorlin syndrome. In xeroderma pigmentosum, recurrent

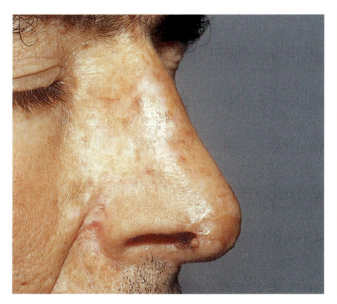

Fig. 8.7. Gorlin syndrome. After surgery

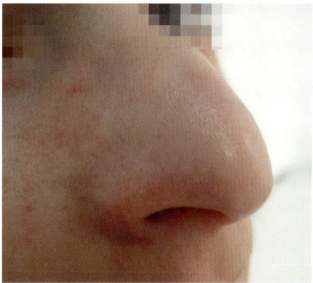

Fig. 8.9. Congenital epidermolysis bullosa

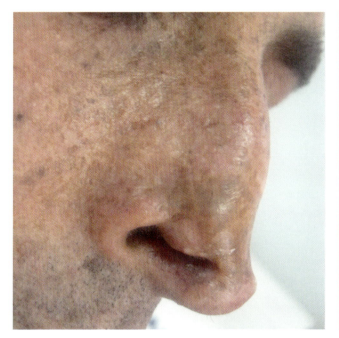

Fig. 8.8. Xeroderma pigmentosum. After skin graft

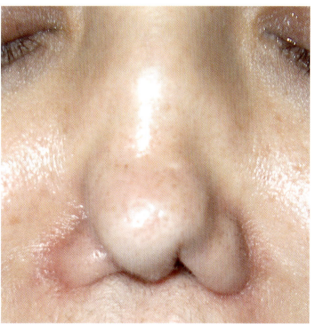

Fig. 8.10. Cicatricial pemphigoid

bullae, secondary skin infections and scars resulting from the application of therapeutic procedures for numerous actinic keratoses may also lead to destruction of the nose. Close monitoring of patients and early therapeutic intervention are important to prevent undesirable deformities.

Recurrent blistering results in scars and may cause the nose to become smaller, especially in the dystrophic form of congenital epidermolysis bullosa (Fig. 8.9). Additionally, atrophy on the nasal skin is remarkable. There is no effective treatment of this disease, and the wide spread skin and mucosal lesions persist during lifetime. Cicatricial pemphigoid sometimes presents with recurrent bullae on the nasal mucosa causing scars and may also damage the septal cartilage resulting with difficulty in breathing (Fig. 8.10). There may be other complications associated with ocular, nasopharyngeal, laryngeal, and anogenital mucosal involvement. Congenital erythropoietic porphyria (Günther's disease) is the most mutilating type of porphyrias in which extreme photosensitivity begins very early in life. Scars resulting from bullous lesions become progressively more prominent on sun-exposed areas, and subcutaneous tissue loss may occur. Besides finger amputation, there may be mutilation of the nasal tip. These serious cosmetic problems may impact the social life of the patient.

Nasal cocaine abuse leads to chronic rhinitis followed by mucosal ulcerations in drug-addicted patients. Septal perforation and depression of the nose due to cartilage necrosis may occur over time. Perforation is due to the vasoconstructive effects of cocaine, traumatic effects of inhalation devices, chemical irritation and secondary infections. Soft as well as hard palate perforations are frequent in these patients. Bleeding, formation of granulation tissue and sinusitis may also occur. It should be remembered that most patients would not admit a history of drug abuse. During the chronic course of mucocutaneous leishmaniasis (espundia), ulceration of the nasal mucosa may enlarge to involve the septum and lead to cartilage destruction. As a result, the nasal bridge and tip may become depressed, but the nasal bone remains intact.

"Saddle nose" is a term used to describe a nose with concave, flattened dorsum and cephalic rotated tip. Nasal cartilage, nasal bone, or both may be depressed in this deformity caused by various diseases, trauma and surgery. Nasal involvement is common in congenital and tertiary syphilis. Early congenital syphilis starts frequently with rhinitis and fissuring around the vestibule, thus the nose is blocked interfering with the child's nursing. Ulcerations develop in persistent and progressive cases resulting in septum perforation, bone destruction and "saddle nose" deformity. Symptoms of late congenital syphilis develop after 5 years of age, but the diagnosis may be delayed until adulthood. Corneal opacities due to interstitial keratitis, Hutchinson's teeth, eighth cranial nerve deafness, "saddle nose" deformity (Figs. 8.11, 8.12)

and rhagades of the lips are characteristic features of this syndrome. The pathognomic lesion of tertiary syphilis is gumma beginning as a subcutaneous nodule which then evolves later to a destructive punched out ulcer. The bony part of the nasal septum may be affected leading to perforation and collapse. Yaws is an endemic treponemal infection with *Treponema pertunea*, which sometimes leads to nasal bone destruction and "saddle nose" deformity in late stages (gangosa). Lepromatous leprosy is another infectious disease which causes "saddle nose" deformity (Fig. 8.13). Necrotizing granulomas in upper and lower respiratory tract are typical findings of Wegener's granulomatosis apart from symmetrical papulonodular lesions on extremities. Most

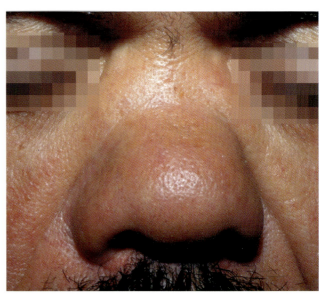

Fig. 8.12. Late congenital syphilis

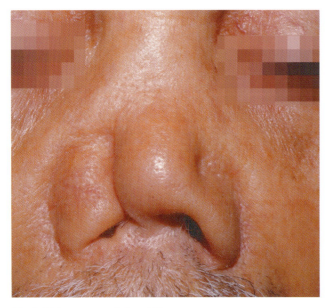

Fig. 8.11. Late congenital syphilis

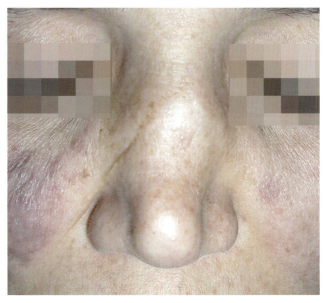

Fig. 8.13. Lepromatous leprosy

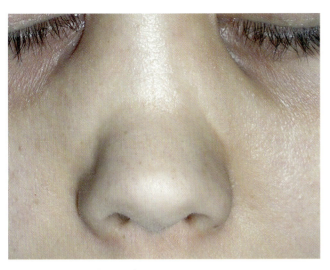

Fig. 8.14. Wegener's granulomatosis

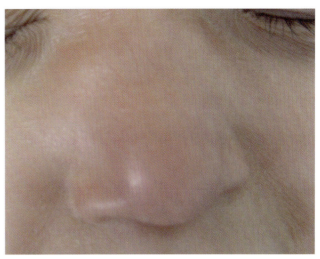

Fig. 8.16. Anhidrotic ectodermal dysplasia

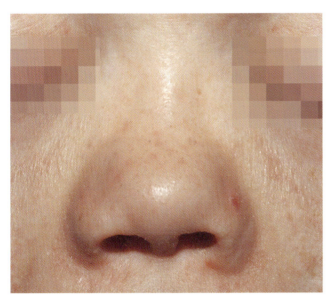

Fig. 8.15. Rothmund-Thomson syndrome

patients also have mucosal involvement and easily ulcerating nasal nodules (Fig. 8.14). Palatal involvement may also develop. As a result of nasal cartilage and bone destruction, "saddle nose" deformity or even necrosis of the nose may emerge. Renal failure due to glomerulonephritis is one of the most important complications. c-ANCA positivity in serological assessment supports the diagnosis. Sarcoidosis may also lead to "saddle nose" deformity by infiltrating the cartilaginous and bony septum, but the patients usually have other well-recognized dermatological signs of the disease. Relapsing polychondritis is a disease affecting the cartilage. Although not as prominent as the ear involvement, the nose may also be affected. Nasal chondritis may lead to cartilage destruction which is replaced by fibrous tissue, resulting in "saddle nose" deformity.

"Saddle nose" deformity may also occur postsurgically especially as a result of the overzealous septorhinoplasty.

Congenital "saddle nose" deformity is seen in some syndromes presenting with facial dysmorphism. Rothmund-Thomson syndrome is characterized by facial erythema, generalized poikiloderma, juvenile cataract, congenital skeletal abnormalities and "saddle nose" deformity which is present from birth (Fig. 8.15). The manifesting features of anhidrotic (hypohidrotic) ectodermal dysplasia are hypo/anhidrosis with hyperpyrexia, fine and sparse hair, dental abnormalities and xerosis. Craniofacial findings are observed as frontal bossing, "saddle nose" with hypoplastic alae, everted thick lips, prominent supraorbital changes, hypoplastic midface and abnormal ears (Fig. 8.16). Most patients are male. Atrophic rhinitis with thick discharge leads to stasis in mucosa and formation of crust, thus there is an increased tendency to infection in paranasal sinuses. Linear ichthyosiform erythroderma following the lines of Blaschko, chondrodysplasia punctata, cataract and short stature may be observed in Conradi-Hünermann-Happle syndrome (X-linked dominant chondrodysplasia punctata), in addition to macrocephaly and "saddle nose" deformity due to nasal bone dysplasia. Cicatricial alopecia, atrophoderma vermiculatum and psoriasiform plaques in intertriginous areas may also be seen. Hurler syndrome is characterized by the impairment of mucopolysaccharide metabolism with "saddle nose" deformity in addition to macrocephaly, thick lips and macroglossia. The most important dermatological feature of prolidase deficiency is chronic ulceration of the lower extremities. Systemic findings include mental retardation and tendency to recurrent sinopulmonary infections. A dysmorphic facial appearance can be observed as "saddle nose", frontal bossing and low hairline.

Cutis laxa develops as a result of elastic fiber damage in dermis and is characterized by redundant and loose skin with a tendency to sagging. The face of these patients shows premature aging (bloodhound-like face). The nose may be hook-like in shape and the philtrum becomes elongated. Goltz syndrome (focal dermal hypoplasia) is characterized by linear atrophic patchy lesions starting from birth, fat herniation, papillomas around the orifices, cicatricial alopecia, nail dystrophia, skeletal defects, ocular abnormalities and a small round facial appearance together with notched nasal wing and wide nasal tip (Fig. 8.17). In Down's syndrome, which is among the most important causes of mental retardation, patients have characteristic flat facies with a small nose and flat nasal bridge, in addition to brachycephaly and short and wide webbed neck (Fig. 8.18). Ear abnormalities may accompany. Short stature, prominent nose and dolicocephalia (thin, narrow head structure) are noted in Bloom's syndrome.

The patients have erythematous telangiectatic patches with a butterfly patern on the face.

In Apert syndrome, craniosynostosis, symmetrical syndactyly and cardiac abnormalities are observed together with beak-like nose and small ears. Intractable acne vulgaris may be seen in these patients. Apart from cardiac abnormalities, mental retardation, short stature and bone defects, dermatological findings such as nevus flammeus and hypertrichosis are observed in Rubinstein-Taybi syndrome. These patients may have a beak-like nose with wide nasal bridge and low level of septum in comparison to ala nasi. 4p-syndrome (Wolf-Hirschhorn syndrome) is associated with the partial deletion of short arm of chromosome 4. In addition to aplasia cutis congenita, some dysmorphic facial features observed are described as "Greek warrior helmet appearance". The nasal root is wide or the nasal tip is beak-like in shape; and microcephaly can be seen in these patients. Bazex-Dupré-Christol syndrome is characterized by multiple basal cell carcinomas of early onset, congenital hypotrichosis, hypohydrosis, profuse milia and follicular atrophoderma. The diagnosis is based on the co-existence of these dermatological features. Some patients show dysmorphic features. Nasal wings may be flat due to hypoplasia (Fig. 8.19). Congenital diffuse hypertrichosis is typical in Ambras syndrome. There is extensive hair on ala nasi and dysmorphic features can be observed such as triangular coarse face, long nose with round tip and anteverted nares.

Leprechaunism (Donohue syndrome) is a disease leading to severe insulin resistance, and manifests with dermatological findings such as generalized lipodystrophy, loose skin, acanthosis nigricans and hirsutism. Patients typically have elf like facies with big, prominent ala nasi, "saddle nose", broad mouth, low set and large ears. Genitalia are large and nipples are prominent. Severe growth retardation begins in

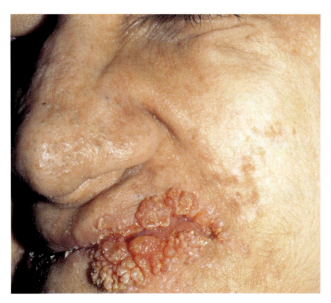

Fig. 8.17. Goltz syndrome

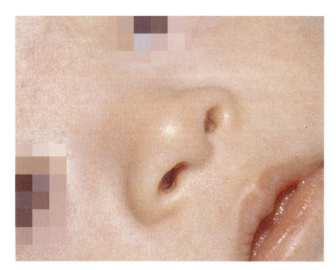

Fig. 8.18. Down's syndrome

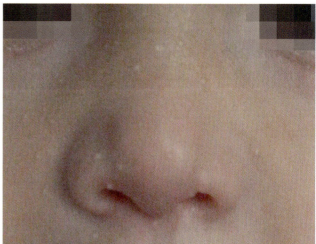

Fig. 8.19. Bazex-Dupré-Christol syndrome

intrauterine life in this disease with poor prognosis. Rabson-Mendenhall syndrome is a disease with milder insulin resistance and prolonged survival when compared to leprechaunism. The phenotype and dysmorphism are similar in some points, but milder in patients with Rabson-Mendenhall syndrome. Dysmorphic features include coarse facies, large ears, prominent forehead, prominent nares and a flattened nasal bridge (Fig. 8.20). Acanthosis nigricans, hirsutism, dental abnormalities, pineal hyperplasia, loss of subcutaneous fat and growth retardation are other clinical features of the disease.

Hyperimmunoglobulinemia-E syndrome is associated with atopiform dermatitis, a coarse facial appearance and nasal structure changes such as widening of the nasal bridge (Fig. 8.21). In this immunodeficiency syndrome, there is an increased tendency to sinopulmonary infections together with very high levels of serum IgE. In patients with Gorlin syndrome, besides scars on the face developed as a result of therapeutic interventions for basal cell carcinomas, a coarse facial appearance, wide nasal root, frontal and parietal protuberance, mandibular prognathy, hypertelorism and strabismus may be observed (Fig. 8.22). In Coffin-Siris syndrome, characterized by absence of nails in fifth fingers and toes, the nose is wide and the nasal bridge is low. In Costello's syndrome, the patients have cutis laxa-like skin. Palmoplantar skin is thickened, and there are papillomas and acrochordons on the face. Coarse facies, thick nasal bridge and inverted nostrils are other morphological features of this disease. Mental retardation and cardiac defects may also occur.

Rhinoscleroma begins insidiously with chronic rhinitis followed by the occurence of a nonulcerating nodule or diffuse sclerotic enlargement. The nose seems like a "hippopotamus nose" (Hebra or tapir nose) in the infiltrative stage due to the involvement of the alar margin and nasal tip. Larynx, trachea and bronchioles may be involved leading to obstruction of airways. Even if long term antibiotic treatment provides some healing, scars and adhesions may occur in the nose and larynx. EEC syndrome is characterized by ectrodactily, ectodermal dysplasia and cleft palate, cleft lip. Lacrimal duct anomalies, genitourinary malformations, mental retardation and facial dysmorphism may be seen in some patients. Wide nasal tip, short philtrum or minor ear abnormalities may accompany. Skin lesions, such as hypopigmented sparse hairs, increased number of melanocytic nevi, xerosis, palmoplantar hyperkeratosis, perioral or intraoral papillomatosis may also be observed. Patients with cardiofacio-cutaneous (CFC) syndrome show multiple congenital anomalies and mental retardation. Failure to thrive, macrocephaly, prominent forehead, bitemporal constriction, absence of eyebrows, hypertelorism, downward-slanting palpebral fissures, low nasal bridge and a bulbous nasal tip are the characteristic findings of this syndrome.

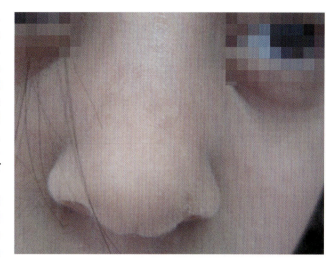

Fig. 8.20. Rabson-Mendenhall syndrome

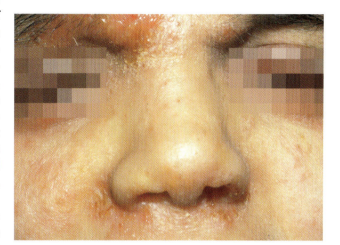

Fig. 8.21. Hyperimmunoglobulinemia-E syndrome

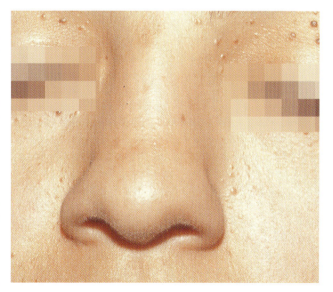

Fig. 8.22. Gorlin syndrome

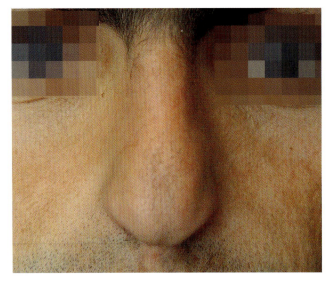

Fig. 8.23. Waardenburg syndrome

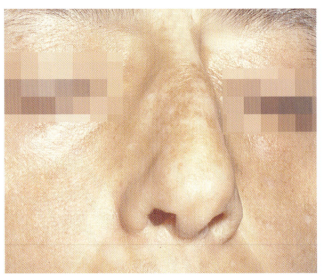

Fig. 8.25. Scleroderma

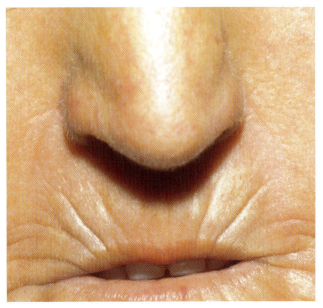

Fig. 8.24. Scleroderma

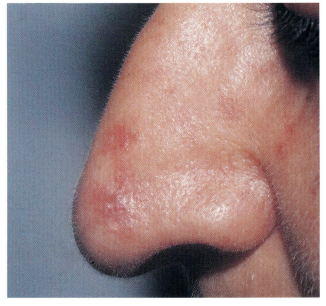

Fig. 8.26. CREST syndrome

The characteristics of trichorhinophalangeal syndrome are nasal structural changes in addition to sparse hair and phalanx abnormalities. In the first type of the disease, the tip of the nose is pear-like in shape and the nasal bridge is broad. In the second type of this disease, microcephaly and mental retardation are noted, and ala nasi is thickened resembling a tent (bulbous nose). Iris heterochromia, dystopia canthorum, congenital sensorineural deafness, abnormal pigmentation of the hair (white forelock) and skin are the signs of Waardenburg syndrome. Melanocyte deficiency in the inner ear is the cause of hearing loss. In this syndrome the nasal root is prominent, short and broad, besides short philtrum (Fig. 8.23). The bridge of the nose is wide due to lateral displacement of the inner canthus of the eyes.

Scleroderma is a collagen vascular disease affecting various internal organs and causing typical facial features. The cheeks are stretched and taut. In addition to the loss of skin lines, the nose is sharp and pinched due to sclerosis (beak-like nose) (Figs. 8.24, 8.25). The limited form of scleroderma, CREST syndrome, shows similar changes on the nose. There are also diffuse telangiectases on the nasal skin (Fig. 8.26). Chronic graft versus host disease, which occurs 3-6 months after bone marrow transplantation, may cause sclerodermoid changes on the face as well as on the extremities. The nose may be hyperpigmented and seem beak-like. In adult patients with porphyria cutanea tarda, the nose becomes smaller due to sclerodermatous changes and atrophy. Kindler syndrome is characterized

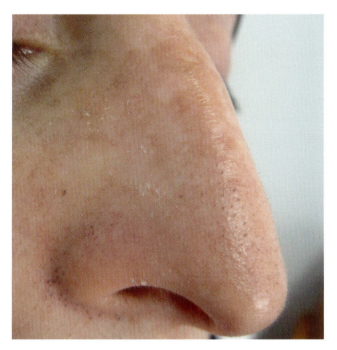

Fig. 8.27. Kindler syndrome

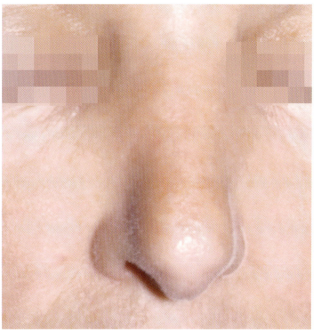

Fig. 8.28. Werner syndrome

by photosensitivity, acral blistering due to minor trauma and progressive sclerotic poikiloderma with atrophy. The nose of the patients becomes smaller and sharpened later on (Fig. 8.27). Morpheaform type of basal cell carcinoma may also cause sharpening of the nose if it involves the nasal tip.

In premature aging syndromes, patients seem older than their actual age, have atrophic skin and some overlapping dysmorphic features. Werner syndrome (adult progeria) manifests with growth retardation, premature atherosclerosis, cataract, characteristic facies and skin changes. Sclerodermoid features are marked in acral regions and may cause atrophy on the face. The face is thin with a pinched expression and a beaked nose, and the ears are inelastic (Fig. 8.28). In Gottron syndrome (acrogeria), besides marked skin atrophy of the hands and feet, there is also atrophy of skin on the tip of the nose. Subcutaneous fat is reduced and the nose is beaked (Fig. 8.29). In Hutchinson-Gilford syndrome (progeria), the skin is thin and wrinkled, hairs are thin and sparse, and nails are thin. The cranium is larger when compared to face. The nose is thin and beak-like, and ears are small without earlobes. Patients with metageria are tall and thin with a tight, bird-like face. The nose is beaked and the eyes are prominent. Poikiloderma and loss of subcutaneous fat accompany. There is subcutaneous fat loss on face with sunken eyes, thin and beak-like nose which all lead to bird-like face in Cockayne syndrome. Patients are typically dwarf. Apart from premature aging syndromes, another disease leading to a thin nose is the vascular type (IV) of Ehlers-Danlos

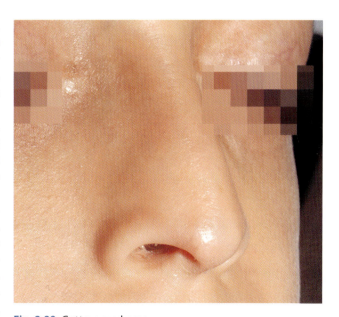

Fig. 8.29. Gottron syndrome

syndrome. The skin is parchment-like, and facial impression of the patients resembles acrogeria.

Transverse nasal line is a common malformation manifesting as a pink line or tiny groove at the upper border of the tip of the nose. It has an embryological origin appearing at the junction of the alar and triangular cartilage. Milia, cysts and comedones show a tendency to localize on this line. It may be confused with the allergic (atopic) salute which is observed at the same location as small transverse lines due to frequent rubbing of the nose in patients with allergic rhinitis.

9 ■ Ulcerative Lesions

Ulceration occurs as a result of dermal or subcutaneous tissue loss, and it usually develops on the base of a tumoral or inflammatory nodule. Thus, an important part of the diseases in this chapter were also mentioned in other chapters of the book. Ulcerative lesions may sometimes develop due to trauma. Lesions as pits on the nose especially occurring at birth are not real ulcerations and they may indicate sinus openings due to dermoid cysts.

A rapidly-developing nodulo-ulcerative lesion on the nose should alert one about the diagnosis of cutaneous leishmaniasis particularly in individuals living in endemic regions. This infestation is seen in all age groups. The nose is an important location for cutaneous leishmaniasis as an unprotected site for sandfly bite. Starting with an erythematous papule at the inoculation site of the protozoal organism (mostly *Leishmania tropica* around the Mediterranean littoral), the lesion enlarges and becomes ulcerated centrally within several months (Figs. 9.1, 9.2). The ulcer is usually covered by a firmly adherent crust showing the typical "tintack" sign which is observed as the projection of underlying horny processes while removing the crust. An erythematous plaque resembling erysipelas may exist around the painless ulceration (Fig. 9.3).

Herpes simplex infection may be seen as a persistent ulceration in intensive care unit patients as well as in patients with AIDS, especially when CD4+ T lymphocyte count is seriously decreased. These lesions with polycyclic margins are usually observed on unusual locations such as the nose and periocular area (Fig. 9.4). Tendency for spontaneous resolution is low, and if not treated with antiviral drugs, it may spread to the central nervous system. Syphilis chancre may occasionally present as a superficial ulceration on the nose. When suspected, dark-field microscopy and serologic evaluation should be performed. Trigeminal neuritis seen in leprosy may result in ulceration on the nose.

As papulonodular lesions of basal cell carcinoma usually ulcerate after a long period, this common tumor represents an important cause of ulceration on the nose (Figs. 9.5, 9.6).

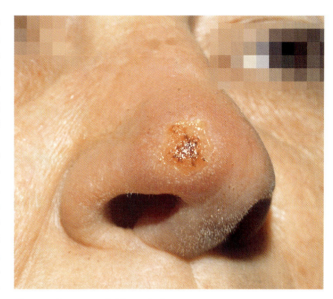

Fig. 9.1. Cutaneous leishmaniasis

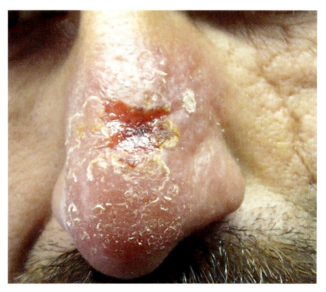

Fig. 9.2. Cutaneous leishmaniasis

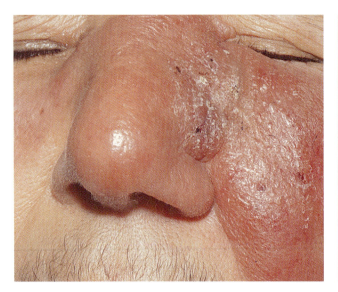

Fig. 9.3. Cutaneous leishmaniasis. Erysipeloid form

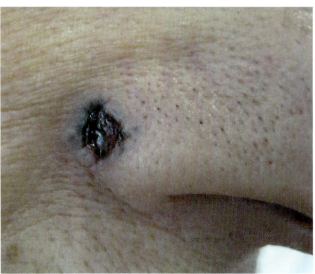

Fig. 9.5. Basal cell carcinoma

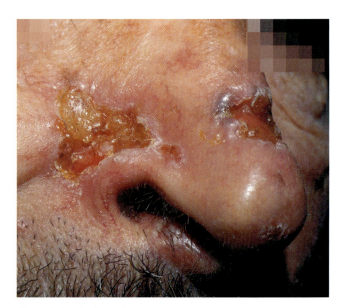

Fig. 9.6. Basal cell carcinoma

Initially, a centrally located superficial ulcer covered by crust is seen which may enlarge within time. The existence of a shiny, pearl-like rolled margin of the tumor is a clue in the diagnosis. In neglected basal cell carcinomas, the ulcer may deepen (rodent ulcer) and sometimes bleed. Furthermore, an unpleasant odour may be a sign of a secondary infection. Squamous cell carcinoma may be located on the nose, but it is not as frequent as basal cell carcinoma. Ulcerated nodular lesion is protuberant, and grows rapidly when compared to basal cell carcinoma (Figs. 9.7, 9.8). The entire surface may be ulcerated and covered by hemorrhagic crust. Squamous cell carcinoma sometimes begins on the nasal vestibule and disseminates to the adjacent skin. Unlike basal cell carcinoma, this tumor may metastasize to local draining lymph nodes and internal organs. Keratoacanthoma is characterized by a rapidly-proliferating nodule in which there is a central crater forming an ulceration covered by an adherent keratotic plug (Figs. 9.9). In contrast to the above mentioned tumors, keratoacanthoma is eventually self-limiting. However, it may cause destruction on the nose and auricle either during the growth phase or regression. During the invasive stage of malignant melanoma, ulcerations occur especially on the nodular parts of the lesions. Amelanotic malignant melanoma may also emerge as

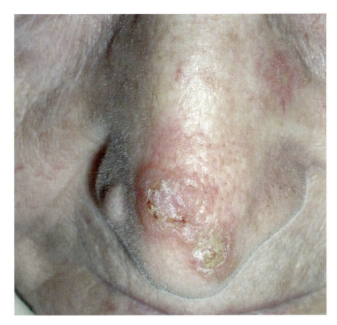

Fig. 9.7. Squamous cell carcinoma

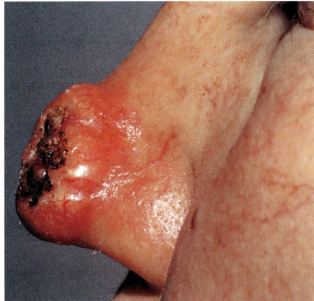

Fig. 9.9. Keratoacanthoma

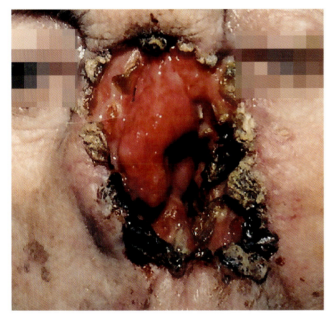

Fig. 9.8. Squamous cell carcinoma

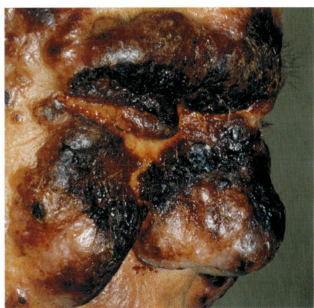

Fig. 9.10. Angiosarcoma

an ulceration without pigmentation. Ulceration is one of the signs of poor prognosis for this tumor.

Purple-coloured, indurated plaques of angiosarcoma may be ulcerated in late stage (Fig. 9.10). Prognosis of this malignancy is poorer after the ulceration has occured. Ulceration may develop especially on large infantile capillary hemangiomas (Fig 6.35). NK (natural killer)/T cell lymphoma is one of the leading causes of destructive nasal ulceration (Figs. 9.11, 9.12). Formerly known as lethal midline granuloma, nasal type of this extra-nodal lymphoma begins with rapidly-growing erythematous and indurated nodules or plaques located on the nose. It may ulcerate in a short time and cause epistaxis, destruction of the bone and nasal obstruction. Sometimes lesions resembling plaques of mycosis fungoides in other areas may accompany. Together with involvement of upper respiratory tract and hemophagocytic syndrome, the prognosis becomes worse. Tumoral lesions of mycosis fungoides may be seen on the nose. Either

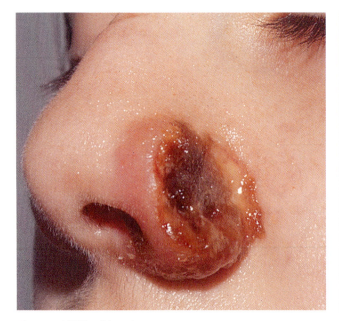

Fig. 9.11. NK/T cell lymphoma

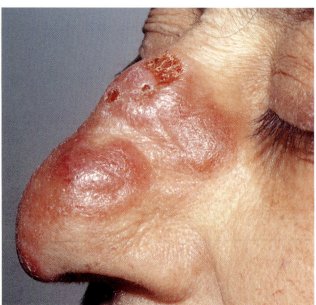

Fig. 9.13. Mycosis fungoides

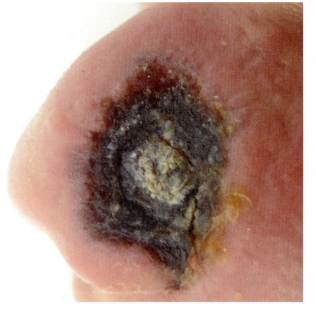

Fig. 9.12. NK/T cell lymphoma

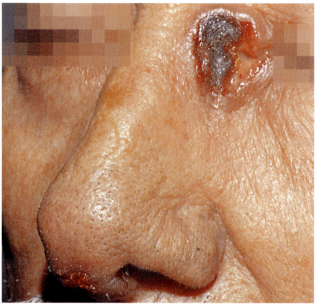

Fig. 9.14. Lymphomatoid papulosis

the entire or a part of the tumor's surface may be ulcerated (Fig. 9.13). The papulonodular and noduloulcerative lesions of lymphomatoid papulosis, a subset of CD30+ lymphoproliferative disorders with good prognosis, may be seen on the nose (Fig. 9.14). The lesions tend to regress spontaneously by leaving scars.

Zygomycosis (mucormycosis) is an opportunistic infection mostly seen in immunocompromised patients. The most common rhinocerebral form of this deep mycosis causes mucosal ulcers in the mouth and on the nose together with ophthalmoplegia, sinusitis and deterioration in general health status. After a while, septum may be perforated and necrosis may emerge in the nose and surrounding tissues. Infection may invade sinuses and central nervous system. Early diagnosis and treatment is important for reducing morbidity and mortality in this disease. Another deep mycosis, histoplasmosis, may also be located on the nose leading to mucosal ulcerations or superficially ulcerated subcutaneous nodules on the skin.

Trigeminal trophic syndrome is a cause of chronic nasal ulceration which occurs as a result of trigeminal nerve damage. Unilateral ulceration starts on the ala nasi after several weeks to years following nerve damage. The nasal tip is typically spared. The ulcer may be deep but does not affect the cartilage. It enlarges slowly to involve the adjacent cheek and upper lip. Ulcers may sometimes be observed on the ears and cornea. Some ulcers involving frontal area may result in triangular frontoparietal alopecia. Most of the cases occur after brain surgery (75%), especially when the Gasser ganglion is removed. Wallenberg syndrome and other cerebrovascular events are other causes of this syndrome. Occasionally, it may result from encephalitis, meningioma, syringobulbia or tabes dorsalis. It is suggested that these ulcers are self-induced, developing on the paresthetic skin due to minor traumas caused by the patients themselves. The chronic ulcer often produces a crescenting shape which can be misdiagnosed as a nonmelanoma skin cancer. Biopsies are often performed to eliminate malignancies. Although surgical reconstruction may be helpful in this ulceration, there is a risk of recurrence.

Ischemic necroses may be seen on the nose in addition to the fingertips and toetips in septic shock. There may be an ulceration starting from the nasal mucosa to involve the upper lip due to nasal cocaine abuse. Pyoderma gangrenosum is a reactive neutrophilic dermatosis that is either idiopathic or it accompanies various systemic diseases and leads to chronic ulcerations. It is located mostly on lower limbs and also on other parts of the body, however, it should be considered in the differential diagnosis of rapidly-growing and long lasting nasal ulcers.

Dermatitis artefacta is a self-inflicted skin lesion. It may coexist with psychiatric diseases or may be seen in individuals who try to get a health report. Hacks, termal sources and

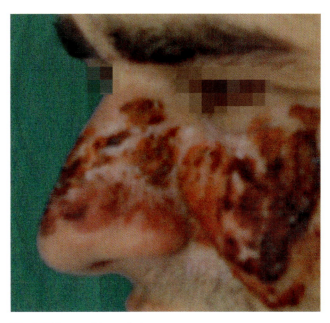

Fig. 9.15. Dermatitis artefacta

irritant chemicals may be used by patients for these aims. Easily reached sites by hands such as the nose are usually affected. Crusted ulcers with clear cut borders and linear geometric pattern suggest the diagnosis (Fig. 9.15). Unlike trigeminal trophic syndrome, functions of trigeminal nerve are normal. Patients do not admit to have manipulated their skin. Besides optimal wound care, occlusive dressings should be used, and the patient should be kept under observation. Healing with the mentioned precautions will support the diagnosis. A substantial number of patients require extensive psychiatric evaluation.

EAR

The Importance from a Dermatological Point of View

Part of the head

An acral region

A periorificial region

A region densely exposed to ultraviolet light

A region open to cold

A region open to trauma

An intertriginous surface

A cartilaginous region

A region with thin skin

A region showing congenital deformity in genodermatoses

Hairy region

C. Baykal and K. Didem Yazganoğlu: *Dermatological Diseases of the Nose and Ears*
DOI: 10.1007/978-3-642-01559-5_10, © Springer-Verlag Berlin Heidelberg 2010

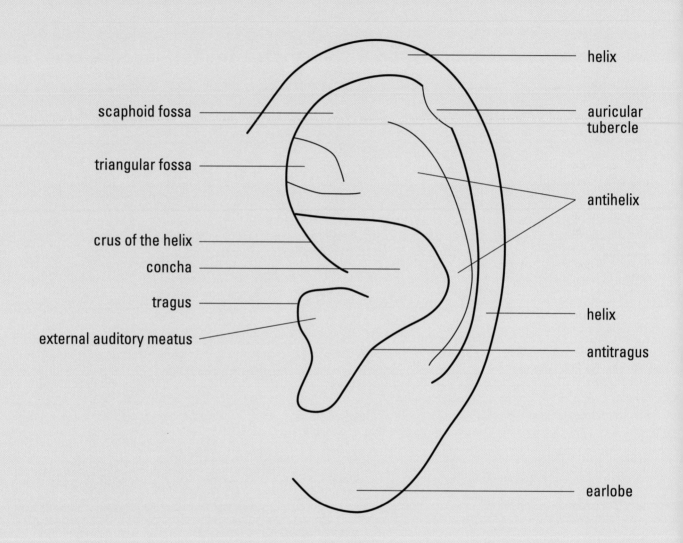

EXTERNAL EAR
[Auricle (pinna) and external auditory canal]

10 ■ Macular Lesions

Pigmentation abnormalities, erythema, purpura and angiomatous macules occuring on the ears have different etiologies. Ochronosis, a disease leading to hyperpigmentation of the ear, presents with bluish black or grey macules (Fig 10.1). It occurs as diffuse hyperpigmentation particularly on the regions above the cartilage such as concha and antihelix, usually during adulthood. Pigment may accumulate in the tympanic membrane, thus the cerumen (earwax) acquires a black colour. This systemic disease can potentially cause cartilage erosion, loss of hearing, tinnitus, and bluish grey scleral pigmentation. Localized argyria occurs due to silver deposit on the skin which manifests as bluish macules at the back side of earlobes due to silver earrings. Argyria may also occur on the ear as a result of intracutaneous application of the acupuncture needles. Pigmentation can appear after a few years, and even more than ten years after contact. Drug eruption associated with systemic agents such as antimalarials and diltiazem may occur as hyperpigmentation clinically similar to ochronosis. Pigmented lichen planus tends to be localized on skin folds and may be observed on the back side of the ear (Fig 10.2). Pityriasis versicolor may occasionally present as well-demarcated hyperpigmented macules covered with fine scales on the ears.

Nevus of Ota, a dermal melanocytic tumor, may cause unilateral hyperpigmentation on the pinna and tympanic membrane in addition to the face and sclera. In Addison's disease which occurs as a result of adrenal insufficiency, a diffuse hyperpigmentation may develop on the ears as well as on many parts of the body. Increased ACTH due to cortisol deficiency is responsible for the pigmentation. In lentigines syndromes, particularly in LEOPARD syndrome and xeroderma pigmentosum, 1-5 mm sized macules of lentigo simplex may occur on the ears as well as on the face (Fig 10.3). Lentigines syndromes may involve various internal organs including the heart. Unilateral lentigines that may sometimes spread from the face towards the ear are observed in segmental lentiginosis. Irregular pigmentation, a sign of photoaging, may also be observed on the ears together with the face and lateral aspects of the neck. Plaques of discoid lupus erythematosus may heal leaving irregular

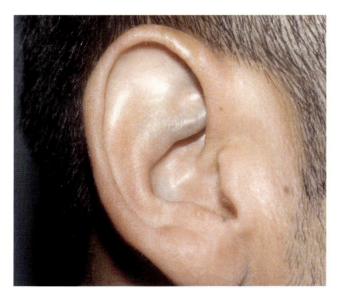

Fig. 10.1. Ochronosis

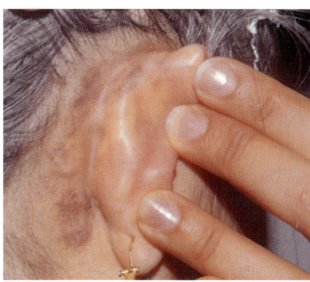

Fig. 10.2. Pigmented lichen planus

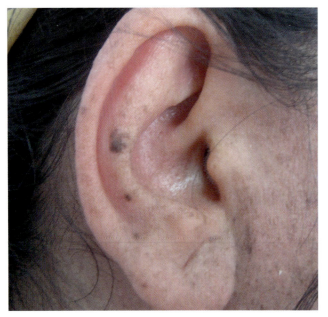

Fig. 10.3. Xeroderma pigmentosum

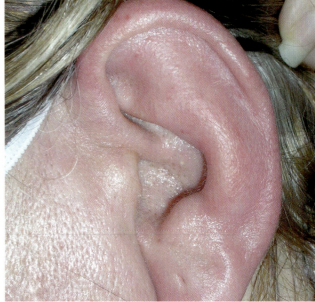

Fig. 10.5. Ara-C ears

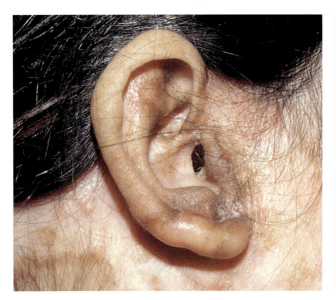

Fig. 10.4. Discoid lupus erythematosus. Dyspigmentation

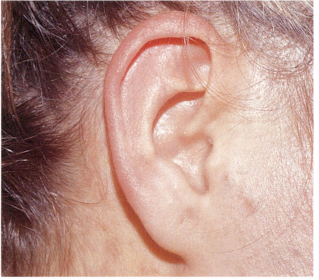

Fig. 10.6. Morbilliform drug eruption

hypo- or hyperpigmentation (Fig 10.4). Vitiligo may cause sharply demarcated depigmented macules on the ears. These lesions have increased vulnerability to sunburn.

While certain disorders may cause an acute erythema on the ear which disappears after a short time, some disorders present with recurrent attacks of ear erythema which may continue for a very long period. Moreover, ear erythema may sometimes be associated with edema. Acute diffuse erythema of the ears may be associated with cytosine arabinoside (cytarabine, ara-C) therapy commonly used in the treatment of acute myeloblastic leukemia (ara-C ears) (Fig. 10.5). Another cutaneous adverse drug reaction with this agent is neutrophilic eccrine hydradenitis which may also involve the ears. However, this reaction is most frequently seen in cases with acute myeloid leukemia and may also develop due to use of other chemotherapeutical agents or some other drugs. Bilateral erythema and edema on the ears may be observed in this dermatosis. Morbilliform (maculopapular) drug eruption frequently involves the face and trunk, and ears may also be erythematous (Fig. 10.6). In the first phase of erythema infectiosum (fifth disease) caused by *Parvovirus B19,* ear involvement may accompany the symmetrical erythema of the cheeks which is also called the "slapped face" appearance. Flushing presents with sudden but transient erythema on the ears together with the face, neck and upper trunk. Skin temparature may also be elavated due to significant vasodilatation during the attacks. Purplish erythema, mild edema and sensitivity on the ears and the palmoplantar area are the initial signs of acute graft versus host disease occurring typically 7 to 21 days after bone marrow transplantation.

Erythromelanosis follicularis faciei appears usually during puberty and presents with symmetrical, well-demarcated erythema of the cheeks (Figs. 10.7, 10.8). Permanent ear erythema may also be seen. Small, horny, follicular papules mostly around the ears accompany erythema. This dermatosis only constitutes a cosmetic problem, and has a chronic course. In rosacea, erythema may also be observed on the ears in addition to the midface. SLE (Figs. 10.9, 10.10) and dermatomyositis (Fig. 10.11) occasionally present with a long-lasting erythema on the ears alongside other parts of the face which is a highly specific region for these collagenoses. Chilblain lupus may also cause permanent erythema on the ears. The erythema of dermatomyositis has a predominantly purplish colour. Transient erythema on the ear together with the cheeks, nose and

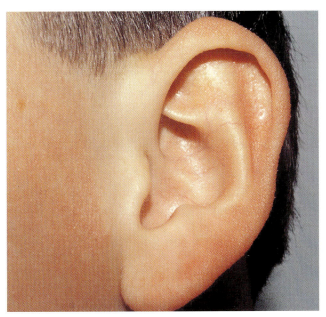

Fig. 10.7. Erythromelanosis follicularis faciei

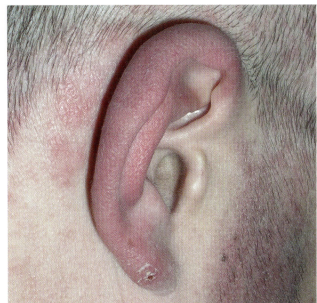

Fig. 10.9. Systemic lupus erythematosus

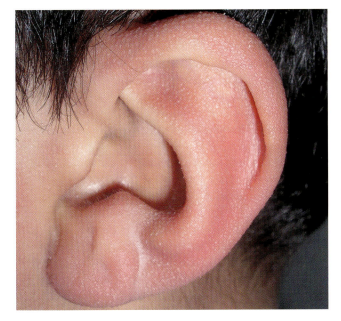

Fig. 10.8. Erythromelanosis follicularis faciei

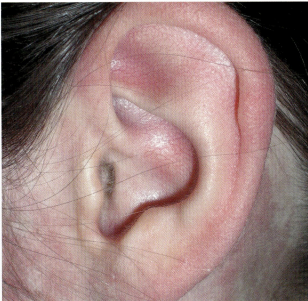

Fig. 10.10. Systemic lupus erythematosus

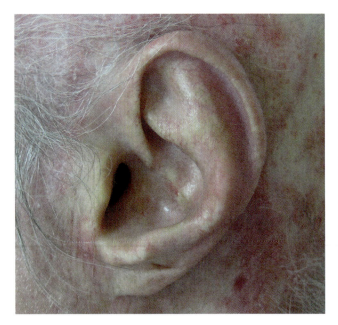

Fig. 10.11. Dermatomyositis

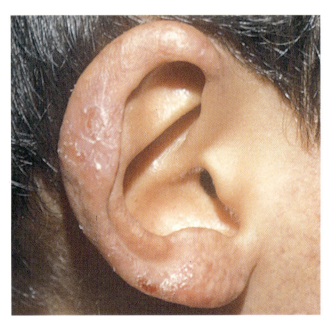

Fig. 10.12. Rothmund-Thomson syndrome

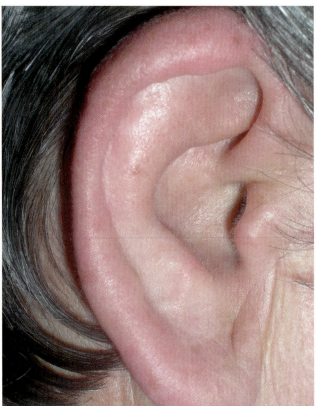

Fig. 10.13. Urticaria

forehead occurring as a result of photosensitivity, are the initial findings of Rothmund-Thomson syndrome. This disease causes poikiloderma in early childhood (Fig. 10.12). In Bloom's syndrome, permanent erythema and telangiectases may develop on the ears. The patients are predisposed to hematological malignancies.

When urticaria and angioedema involve the ears, pinna is typically erythematous and swollen due to dermal or subcutaneous edema (Fig. 10.13). These patients may complain of severe pruritus. While urticarial plaques resolve in a short time, new lesions may occur on other parts of the body. Cellulitis may present with a tender erythematous patch associated with edema. Auricular involvement is mostly unilateral in this bacterial infection which may develop due to ear piercing. Patients also have systemic symptoms such as fever and chills. It may start from the ears and spread towards the surrounding skin. Sometimes cellulitis may develop in the setting of seborrheic dermatitis. Systemic antibiotics are the mainstay of the treatment. As a result of the injury in the lymphatics of the external ear, recurrent attacks of cellulitis may develop on the ears and lead to thickening of the overlying skin.

Relapsing polychondritis is an autoimmune disease involving multiple cartilaginous structures of the body and is frequently seen on the ears (Figs. 10.14, 10.15). Severe inflammation and pain accompany bright red ear erythema during long lasting attacks. While the areas over the cartilage tissue are involved in both ears, earlobes remain unaffected. Nonerosive inflammatory polyarthritis and ocular inflammation are common systemic findings. Since it may cause complications such as asphyxia secondary to tracheal cartilage involvement, and aneurysm secondary to major vessel involvement, a multidisciplinary approach is required. In patients with MAGIC syndrome, Behçet's disease and relapsing polychondritis coexist. Infectious perichondritis or chondritis is a bacterial infection occurring on the ear perichondrium (perichondritis) or cartilage (chondritis) which develops secondary to trauma such as laceration of the auricle, surgery, frostbite, burns or high piercing of the cartilage. It is mostly unilateral. The skin may be erythematous, edematous and painful. *Pseudomonas aeruginosa* is responsible for the chondritis especially if it develops after ear piercing. Concomitant use of systemic antibiotics with incision and drainage may be required. The infection usually regresses within 1 to 3 months, however it may sometimes result in permanent ear deformity.

Erythromelalgia is typically characterized by paroxysmal episodes of burning sensation or pain, redness and increased temperature on the hands and feet. It may occasionally be limited to the ears. Both ears may be completely erythematous and edematous. The symptoms are typically aggravated by the increased environmental temperature and exercise, and relieved by cooling. The disease may be idiopathic (primary) or associated with certain systemic diseases (secondary) such as SLE, myeloproliferative diseases and hypertension, and also medication. The red ear syndrome is characterized by pain in and around the ear associated with attacks of erythema and ipsilateral burning sensation in the ear. Headache can occur for a period of approximately one hour. The idiopathic form that is usually associated with migraine is commonly encountered in young individuals. The secondary form of red ear syndrome is observed at older ages. It is mostly associated with disorders of the upper cervical region. Sweet's syndrome (acute febril neutrophilic dermatosis) develops idiopathic or reactively in the setting of systemic infections, malignancies and inflammatory bowel diseases, and presents with multiple well-demarcated erythematous plaques on the face, upper trunk and extremities. This dermatosis may occasionaly involve the ears bilaterally leading to acute erythema, edema and pain.

Purpura secondary to trauma can easily occur on the ears (Fig. 10.16). Children exposed to domestic violence may have petechia or ecchymoses on the external ear or retroauricular area. In infantile (acute) hemorrhagic edema, mostly observed in children aged 4 months to 2 years, purpura on the ear may accompany the typical edematous purpuric plaques of the cheeks (Fig. 10.17). This idiopathic minor vessel vasculitis may also affect the lower extremities, scrotum and umbilicus. A mild increase in body temperature may be observed; but the patient's overall general state tends to be fine. Lesions spontaneously regress within 3 weeks, and recurrence is rare. Purpuric macules are observed occasionally on the pinna as well as lower extremities during the course of Henoch-Schönlein

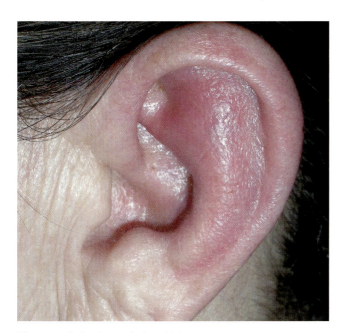

Fig. 10.14. Relapsing polychondritis

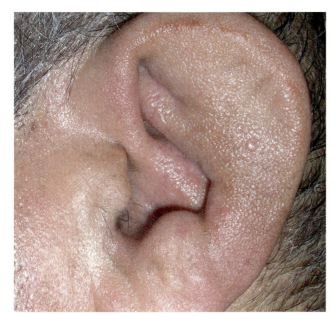

Fig. 10.15. Relapsing polychondritis

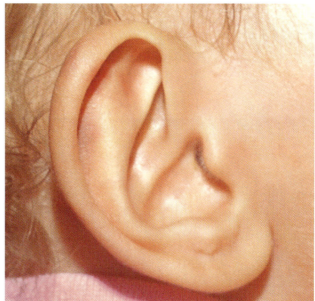

Fig. 10.16. Purpura secondary to trauma

purpura. This vasculitis may also affect the kidneys, gastrointestinal system and the joints, and has a high rate of recurrence. Another systemic disease, which may lead to purpura on the ears, is idiopathic thrombocytopenic purpura. Mucosal hemorrhages may accompany this condition. In cryoglobulinemia, purpura may occur on the ear helix and nose together with the acral parts of the hands and feet. Lesions may be tender or painful. This cold dermatosis may also cause ulcers and necrotic lesions in addition to purpura.

Port-wine-stain type of nevus flammeus may cause a well-demarcated angiomatous macule on the ear, but this is not as common as it is seen on the nose (Fig. 10.18). Red patches may extend to the cheek and neck. Involvement is usually unilateral, and the ear with the hemangioma may be larger compared to the other one.

Telangiectases are thin linear lesions, resulting from the dilatation of the venules on papillary dermis and are usually located on the antihelix region of the ear. Chronic ultraviolet light damage is the most important reason for ear telangiectases observed in adult patients (Figs. 10.19, 10.20). In addition, it may develop secondarily in some genodermatoses. Ataxia telangiectasia, characterized by cerebellar ataxia and immunodeficiency, presents with diffuse fine telangiectases on the ears together with the eyes and face

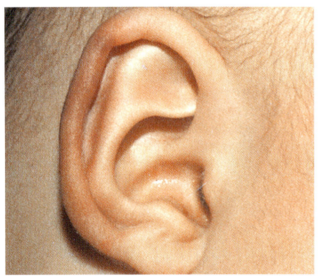

Fig. 10.17. Infantile hemorrhagic edema

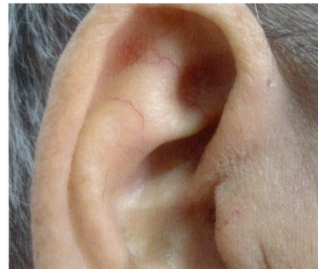

Fig. 10.19. Chronic ultraviolet light damage

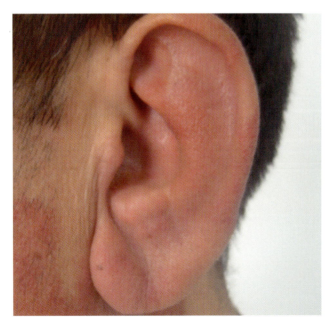

Fig. 10.18. Nevus flammeus. Port-wine-stain

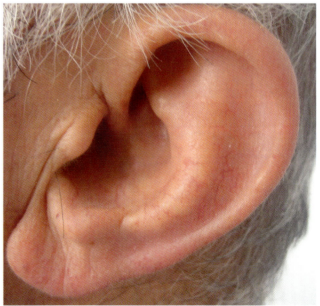

Fig. 10.20. Chronic ultraviolet light damage

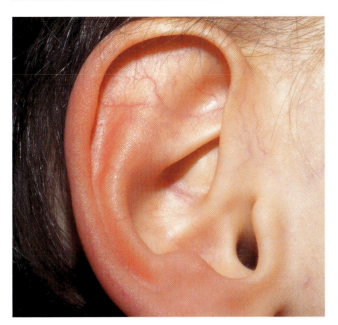

Fig. 10.21. Ataxia telangiectasia

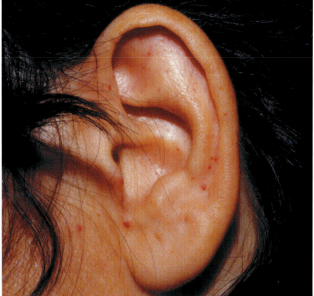

Fig. 10.22. Rendu-Osler-Weber syndrome

typically starting in the childhood (Fig. 10.21). The lesions may become more prominent over time. In Rendu-Osler-Weber syndrome, telangiectases on the external ear typically accompany the telangiectases of the mucosa or other parts of the skin in the form of 3-10 mm wide macules or nonpulsatile, bright red papules (Fig. 10.22). In this genodermatosis, telangiectases may also be observed on the tympanic membrane.

Telangiectases on the external auditory canal may be seen in connective tissue disorders like scleroderma.

11 ■ Vesiculobullous and Pustular Lesions

The most important causes of the vesiculobullous and pustular lesions located on the ear include viral and bacterial infections, immunobullous dermatoses, vasculitis and diseases triggered by physical factors. Pressure-related bullae develop easily on the ears. Serous, opaque bullae occurring due to exposure to cold below the freezing point may also be located on this region. This condition is called frostbite and may be accompanied by severe pain. Ethyl chloride sprays used as an anesthetic in the procedure of ear piercing may also cause a similar clinical picture.

In varicella, primary *Varicella zoster virus* infection mainly observed in children, 2 to 3 mm sized, itchy vesicles with central umbilication may be located on the ears as well as on the trunk, scalp and the face (Fig. 11.1). These lesions crust over and heal with scars. Vesicles located on an erythematous base limited to a single ear (helix, antihelix, earlobe, concha, external auditory canal and tympanic membrane) accompanied by pain spreading to the tonsillar region are the findings of zona oticus, which is also called Ramsay-Hunt syndrome (Fig. 11.2). This secondary *Varicella zoster virus* infection is mostly observed in adults, and its severity is variable. While it sometimes only involves ears, occasionally function of the 7th and 8th cranial nerves can be impaired. Sensory and motor components of nervus facialis are affected, and unilateral peripheral facial paralysis occurring 1-2 weeks after the rash precludes the patient from closing their eye. Systemic symptoms including impairment of taste secondary to involvement of 7th cranial nerve and tinnitus, vertigo and rarely sensorineural hearing loss secondary to the involvement of the 8th cranial nerve may accompany this condition. In this form of herpes zoster, early systemic antiviral treatment should be instituted to prevent the complications.

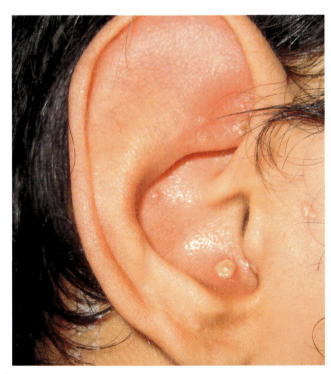

Fig. 11.1. Varicella

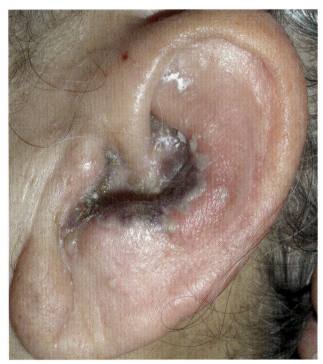

Fig. 11.2. Ramsay-Hunt syndrome (Zona oticus)

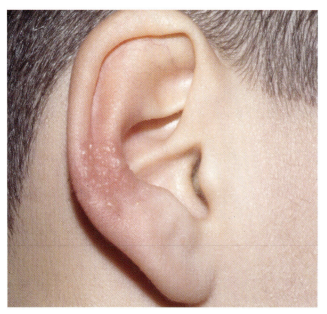

Fig. 11.3. Herpes simplex infection

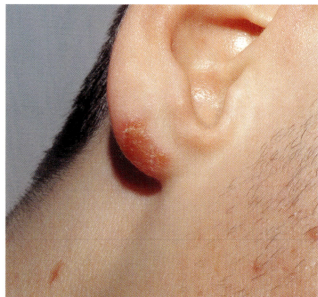

Fig. 11.4. Impetigo

Grouped vesiculopustular lesions of the herpes simplex infection that cause sensation of burning and paresthesiae early on may rarely be located on the ear (Fig. 11.3). Herpes gladiatorum, a form of this viral infection observed in wrestlers, may affect the sides of the face and ears. Generally, a wrestler with labial herpes may infect his competitor on different sites of his body via inoculation during the competition. Eczema herpeticum is a widespread vesicular eruption caused by *Herpes simplex virus,* mostly in individuals with atopic dermatitis. Umbilicated vesicles some of which are hemorrhagic may arise on the face and ears. Exudation and crusting on eroded lesions may be prominent. In addition, fever and other systemic symptoms may be present.

Superficial vesiculobullous lesions of impetigo caused by staphylococci or streptococci may be located on the ears. Since lesions crust after a short while, intact bullae are not seen frequently (Fig. 11.4). Concomitant regional lymphadenopathy may be present. This type of pyoderma is commonly observed in children, but may also spread to adults after close contact. A rare complication of streptococcal impetigo is glomerulonephritis. Impetigo may occur on intact skin. It may also be seen as a secondary infection in ear eczema (secondary impetiginization). Staphylococcal folliculitis may occasionally manifest as pustules on the ear (Fig. 11.5). Furuncle of the ears is most commonly located at the junction between tragus and the anterior crus of the helix. Cutaneous anthrax may rarely be located on the ears depending on the inoculation site of *Bacillus anthracis.* It spreads from cattles to humans and may occur as an occupational disease in people dealing with stockbreeding. It starts with a pustule at the site of inoculation, then spread peripharily and evolve to bullae and hemorrhagia over time. After a while, a black, necrotic crust occurs. Edema

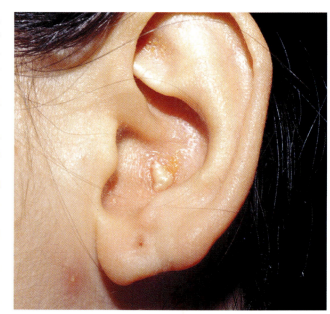

Fig. 11.5. Folliculitis

particularly on the head and neck region, and sepsis are the rare complications of cutaneous anthrax. Favorable response to antibiotic treatment is achieved in most cases. Lesions generally heal without scars.

External otitis (swimmer's ear) is an infection of soft tissues of the external ear and surrounding structures caused by pseudomonas in individuals, who are otherwise healthy. Malignant external otitis is again caused by pseudomonas particularly in elderly, diabetic patients, HIV infected patients and immunosuppressed patients. Both conditions may lead to development of pustular lesions (Fig. 11.6). The acidic nature of the cerumen formed by the apocrine and sebaceous glands in the external auditory canal exhibits a protective effect by inhibiting gram-negative bacteria. Impairment of this balance during swimming facilitates external otitis. External otitis may also occur following surgery. In those with an underlying systemic disease mucormycosis and aspergillosis may also lead to malignant external otitis. Erythema, edema, maceration and severe pain are other symptoms of external otitis. A moist waste product may accumulate in the external auditory canal due to serous discharge. All the symptoms are more severe in malignant external otitis. Pus formation is intense and may cause a bad odour. Ear pain is particularly disturbing at night. Infection may persist for weeks or months. Malignant external otitis should be treated early with appropriate antibiotics, since it may result in severe complications such as cartilage necrosis, osteomyelitis of the head bones, facial nerve paralysis or sepsis.

Pemphigus vulgaris rarely involves the ear, and intact bullae on this location are unusual (Fig. 11.7). Erosions may also be seen on the external auditory canal. Ear symptoms include auditory canal obstruction and pain. Auricular involvement is relatively frequent in linear IgA dermatosis. The base of the serous bullae is erythematous or urticarial (Figs. 11.8, 11.9). In dermatitis herpetiformis, usually excoriated, pruritic vesicles

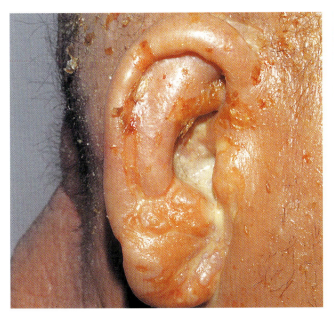

Fig. 11.6. Malignant external otitis (in a patient with Sezary syndrome)

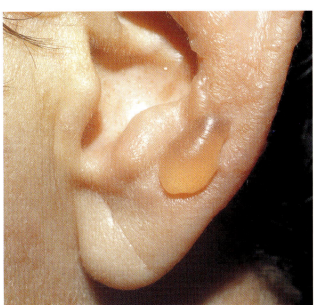

Fig. 11.8. Linear IgA dermatosis

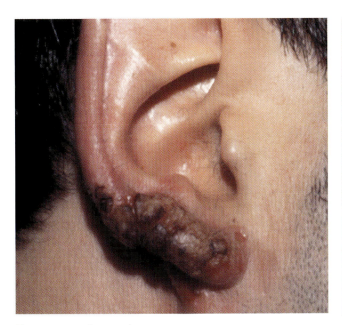

Fig. 11.7. Pemphigus vulgaris

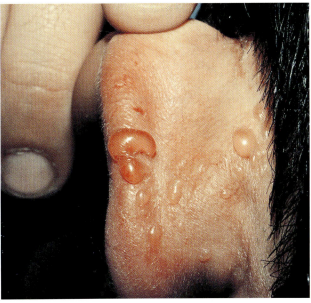

Fig. 11.9. Linear IgA dermatosis

are seen on the ears. While bullous pemphigoid is infrequently encountered on the ear, milia may develop after healing of the bullous lesions. Cicatricial pemphigoid may involve the ears in addition to other cutaneous sites and mucosal surfaces or occasionally it may only be localized on the ears (Fig. 11.10). This disease may involve the external ear together with the middle ear and the tympanic membrane, and can cause loss of hearing due to scarring. In lichen planus pemphigoides, disseminated bullous lesions may also be observed on the ears (Fig. 11.11). Diagnosis of immunobullous dermatoses is mostly established by histopathology and direct immunofluorescence. Ear is not a preferred site for biopsy, and biopsies are generally taken from lesions on other sites of the body.

In congenital epidermolysis bullosa, recurrent bullae may occur on the ears starting in the new born period, especially depending on the sleeping position. Over time, severe milia and scars may develop (Fig. 11.12). Although rare, hemorrhagic bullae may be observed on the ears in cases of vasculitis. In Wegener's granulomatosis, bullae may occur on the ears as well as on different parts of the body (Fig. 11.13). Juvenile spring eruption, a specific form of polymorphic light eruption, frequently occurs in boys between 5 to 12 years of age,

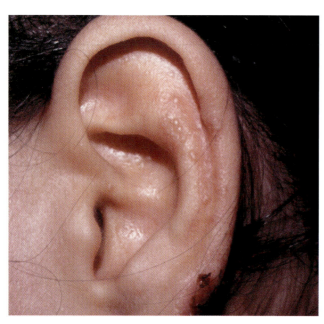

Fig. 11.10. Cicatricial pemphigoid

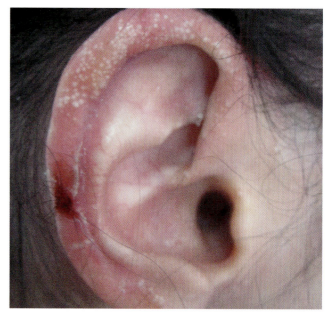

Fig. 11.12. Congenital epidermolysis bullosa

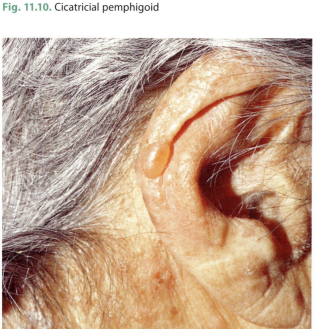

Fig. 11.11. Lichen planus pemphigoides

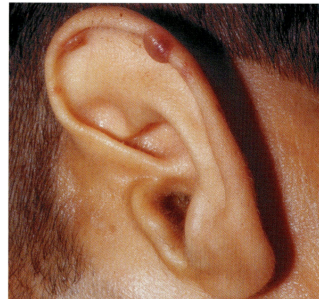

Fig. 11.13. Wegener's granulomatosis

11 Vesiculobullous and Pustular Lesions

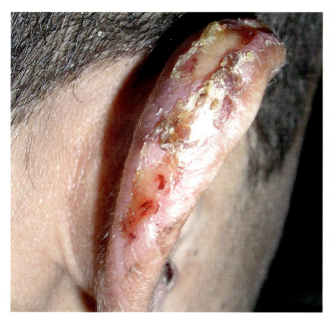

Fig. 11.14. Hydroa vacciniforme

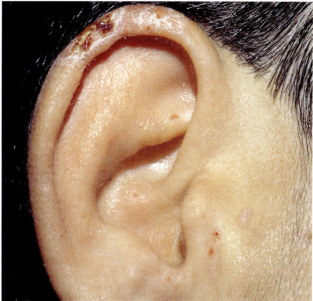

Fig. 11.16. Porphyria cutanea tarda

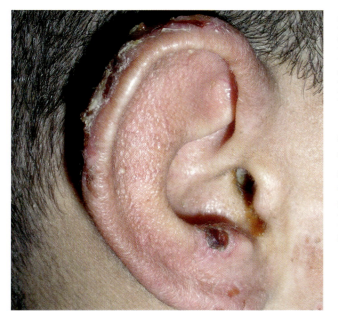

Fig. 11.15. Hydroa vacciniforme

and typically in the form of papules and vesicles on the ear helix. It may cause mild pruritus and pain. Lesions tend to improve within 2 weeks without leaving scars. In hydroa vacciniforme, the papules, vesicles and bullae recurring mostly on the upper part of the auricle may cause necrosis and scars (Figs. 11.14, 11.15). Actinic prurigo manifests with papules and vesicles on sun-exposed areas that gradually turn into eczematous lesions. In porphyria cutanea tarda, excess porhyrins results in the development of bullae on the ears as well as the face (Fig. 11.16). Recurrent lesions usually heal with scars. Paroxysmal nocturnal hemoglobinuria is an acquired clonal hematological disease characterized by hemoglobinuria and thrombosis. Purpura and hemorrhagic bullae may sometimes be observed on the ears.

Hydradenitis suppurativa is a chronic inflammatory disease affecting the hair follicles and apocrine glands. In addition to its primary localization on the axillary and anogenital areas, it may lead to recurrent abscess-like lesions on the retroauricular area, earlobe and external auditory canal in severe cases. These ear lesions may sometimes lead to complications such as otitis media, external otitis and even hearing loss.

12 ■ Eczematous and Squamous Lesions

In many inflammatory dermatoses commonly seen in dermatological practice, eczematous or squamous lesions may be observed on the ears. However, diseases with different etiologies may also cause a similar picture. Seborrheic dermatitis frequently involves retroauricular area and sometimes the external ear, usually bilaterally (Fig. 12.1). Lesions located on the back side of the ear may exhibit a chronic course in childhood. In this region, poorly demarcated, pink, red or yellowish brown-coloured, moist patches are frequently observed (Figs. 12.2, 12.3). The patches are covered with yellow, greasy scales and show fissures. Seborrheic dermatitis in intertriginous areas may be pruritic. Rarely, a clinical picture consisting of erythema, eroded areas, greasy scales, weeping and crusts covering the whole external ear may be observed (Fig. 12.4). Scales may accumulate in the external auditory canal and cause itching. Superimposed secondary bacterial infections may lead to a bad odour. Frequent recurrence of this disease despite achievement of a good initial

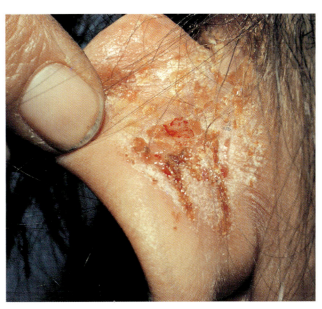

Fig. 12.2. Seborrheic dermatitis

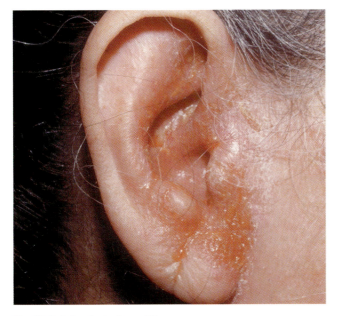

Fig. 12.1. Seborrheic dermatitis

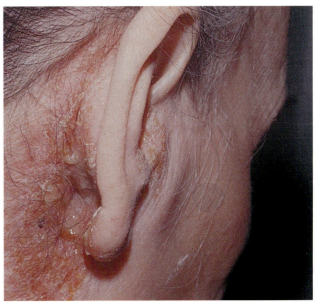

Fig. 12.3. Seborrheic dermatitis

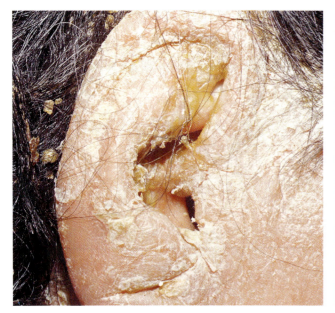

Fig. 12.4. Seborrheic dermatitis

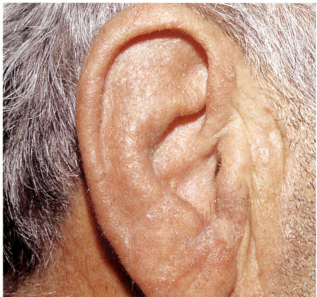

Fig. 12.5. Tinea faciei

therapeutic response may cause patients to give up using drugs after a while.

Langerhans cell histiocytosis may cause a clinical picture on the ear similar to seborrheic dermatitis but is resistant to topical therapies. This disease is mostly observed in children and has a chronic course. While erosion and exudation may occur on the external auditory canal, moisturization, erosion and scales can be observed on the retroauricular region. Petechiae may be prominent on these patches. Lesions may also occur on the other intertriginous areas of the body. Prognosis depends on the visceral involvement. Dermatophytoses may lead to scaling and itching on the external auditory canal. The border of the lesions may be ill-defined in this region. On the other hand, erythematous, squamous, well-demarcated, dry plaques of tinea faciei may spread from other parts of the face to the external ear (Fig. 12.5). In case of suspected fungal infection, native preparation should be performed. Dermatophyte infections respond well to antifungal treatment and heal without scars.

Allergic eczematous contact dermatitis may develop on the ear due to various reasons (Figs. 12.6-12.8). Eczema caused by earrings is a common problem in women. It usually occurs due to earrings containing nickel. However, it should be remembered that golden earrings may also contain nickel at their attachment site. Ill-defined, erythematous, squamous and sometimes weeping lesions mostly start from the earlobe and spread to other parts of the ear and to the adjacent skin. It is sometimes hard to differentiate these lesions from seborrheic dermatitis. Mobile phones containing nickel and chromium may cause eczema particularly at the site where the phone contacts. Eczema may involve other body regions that have been exposed to relevant metals.

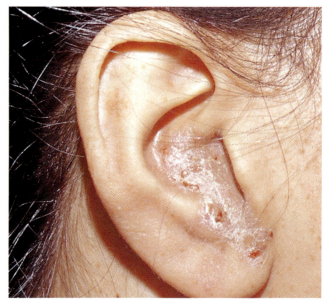

Fig. 12.6. Allergic eczematous contact dermatitis

After the diagnosis is confirmed by a patch test, contact with nickel should be avoided. If no precautions are taken, pruritic lesions may result in lichenification. Creams and drops containing substances such as gentamycin and neomycin which are commonly used for the treatment of external otitis are among the significant causes of ear eczema. Allergic eczematous contact dermatitis may develop due to hair dyes (paraphenylenediamine), and it commonly affects the ear as well as the scalp and the neck. Other than these, many topical drugs and chemical agents may also cause ear eczema in susceptible individuals. Contact dermatitis may occur at the

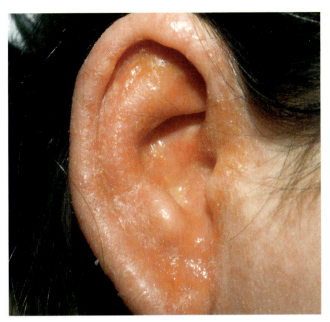

Fig. 12.7. Allergic eczematous contact dermatitis

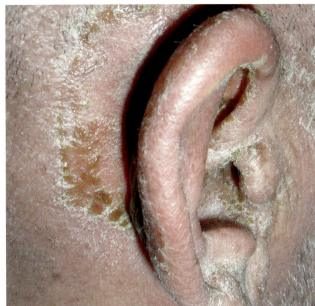

Fig. 12.9. Eczematous drug reaction

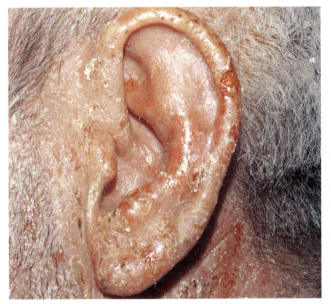

Fig. 12.8. Allergic eczematous contact dermatitis

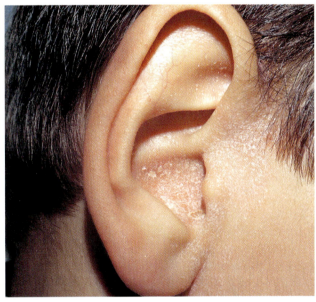

Fig. 12.10. Atopic dermatitis

back of the ear due to frames of glasses. Contact dermatitis generally responds well to topical corticosteroid treatment. However, this disease may recur upon re-exposure to the same relevant agent. Diffuse eczematous drug reactions may involve the ear as well as other parts of the body (Fig. 12.9). Presence of chronic eczematous lesions on the external ear and earlobe rhagade (fissure) are typical for atopic dermatitis (Figs. 12.10-12.12). Earlobe rhagades are also among the various specific diagnostic criteria for this disease. The ear may have a lichenified appearance at the late stage of atopic dermatitis (Fig. 12.13). It may be necessary to use topical cor-

ticosteroids for the treatment of eczematous lesions. In hyperimmunoglobulinemia-E syndrome, treatment-resistant eczematous lesions may occur on the ears. Intertrigo which is usually observed on the skin folds of obese people may sometimes manifest as erythema, maceration and fissures on the retroauricular area.

Squamous plaques on eroded base may develop on the ear due to pemphigus foliaceus. If suspected, investigations for immunobullous dermatoses including Tzanck cytology should be performed. Follicular mucinosis (alopecia mucinosa) manifests itself as erythematous and sometimes

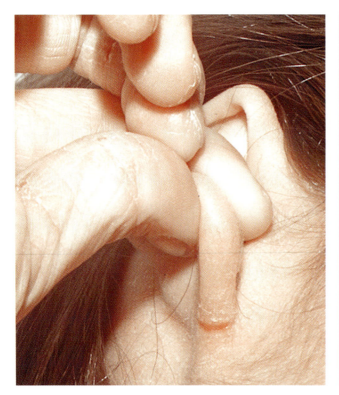

Fig. 12.11. Atopic dermatitis. Earlobe rhagade

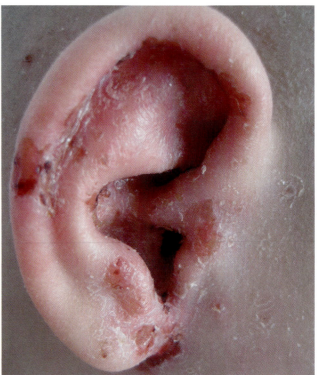

Fig. 12.13. Atopic dermatitis

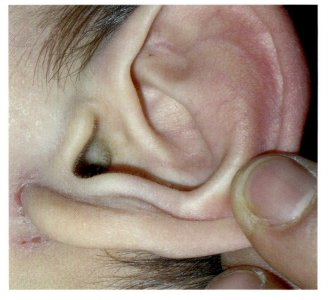

Fig. 12.12. Atopic dermatitis. Earlobe rhagade

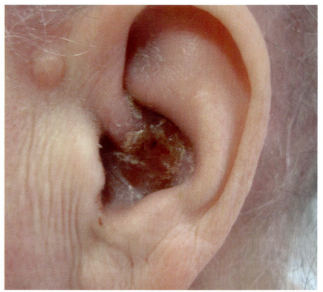

Fig. 12.14. Follicular mucinosis

eczema-like plaques. (Fig. 12.14). Hair loss may occur on the lesion as a result of mucin accumulation in hair follicles. Follicular orifices are prominent and there may be follicular papules. The ear is one of the most commonly affected areas. This form of cutaneous mucinosis may be associated with cutaneous lymphomas such as mycosis fungoides and Sezary syndrome or may be idiopathic. The prognosis varies depending on the concomitant disease. Idiopathic forms may regress spontaneously. Pediculosis capitis leads to severe pruritus on the nape. Excoriation, crusts and secondary eczematization may occur on the ears as well as the nape as a result of host's reaction to the bites of the lice. The presence of parasite eggs (nits) on the hairs is diagnostic. Symmetrical ear involvement with well-demarcated, eroded, scaly or crusted plaques may be seen in acrodermatitis enteropathica.

Psoriasis vulgaris may affect the ear in approximately 20% of patients (Figs. 12.15-12.17). There may be well-demarcated, erythematous, squamous and dry plaques anywhere

12 Eczematous and Squamous Lesions

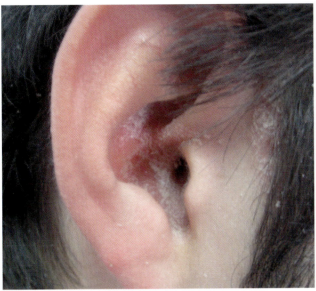

Fig. 12.15. Psoriasis vulgaris

Fig. 12.17. Psoriasis vulgaris

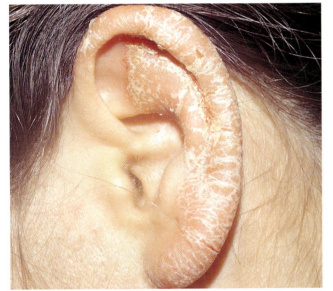

Fig. 12.16. Psoriasis vulgaris

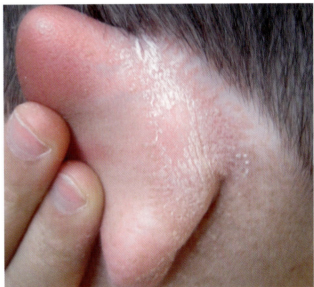

Fig. 12.18. Pityriasis rubra pilaris

on the ear. A large amount of scales may accumulate in the external auditory canal. The ear should be protected against traumas in order to prevent the Koebner effect. During long term topical corticosteroid treatment for ear lesions, it should be remembered that the ear skin is thin, therefore side effects such as atrophy may easily develop especially with potent preparations. In cases of psoriasis inversa which is the form of the disease involving the intertriginous regions like the retroauricular area, maceration and fissures may be prominent on erythematous plaques rather than thick scales. It is frequently misdiagnosed as seborrheic dermatitis in the absence of associated typical lesions. Pityriasis rubra pilaris may cause scaling on the ear as well as redness and fine scales on the face (Fig. 12.18). Since the clinical features on the auricle is not typical, the diagnosis can be established by the presence of other lesions of the disease. The rash of pityriasis rosea with collarate-like scales occasionally involves face and ears (Fig. 12.19).

Discoid lupus erythematosus is commonly observed on the ear, since it is a region highly exposed to ultraviolet light. It mostly occurs on the earlobe, helix and choncae as one or a few well-demarcated, round, oval or irregularly-shaped erythematous plaques with a slightly raised edge and adherent white scales (Figs. 12.20, 12.21). Plaques may be associated

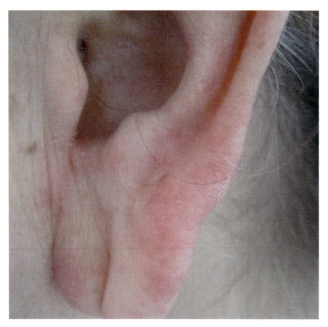

Fig. 12.19. Pityriasis rosea

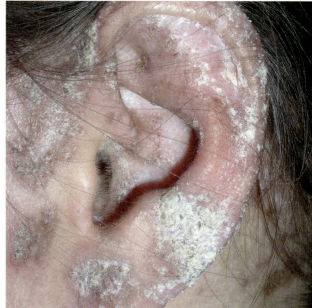

Fig. 12.21. Discoid lupus erythematosus

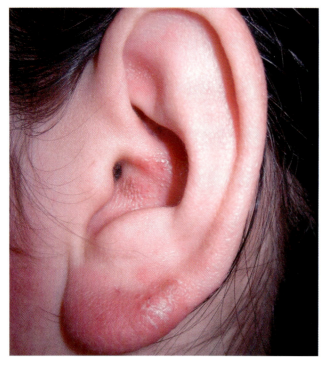

Fig. 12.20. Discoid lupus erythematosus

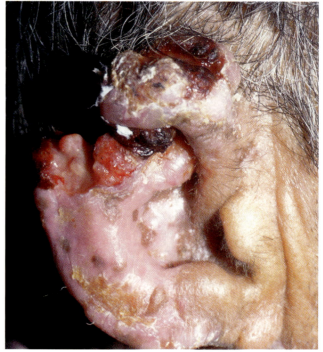

Fig. 12.22. Squamous cell carcinoma developing on the scar of discoid lupus erythematosus

with initial lesions such as small, comedo-like follicular plugs. Occasionally, ulceration may develop on the plaques. Lesions spread peripherally leaving atrophic scars and dyspigmentation. The presence of small scars on the concha is typical. Although histopathological examination has a significant role in the diagnosis of discoid lupus erythematosus, biopsy from the regions other than ears is preferable. Treatment in combination with protection against sun mostly provides favorable results, however the disease may recur in other areas. Since squamous cell carcinoma may occasionally develop on scars of discoid lupus erythematosus, patients sould be followed up even after the skin lesions settle (Fig. 12.22).

12 Eczematous and Squamous Lesions

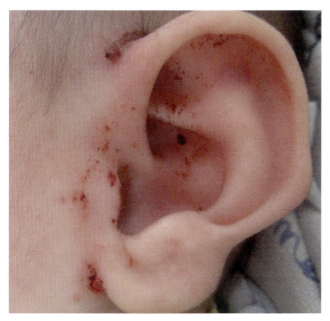

Fig. 12.23. Wiskott-Aldrich syndrome

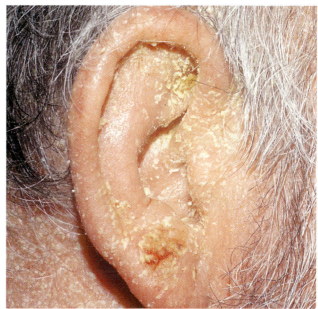

Fig. 12.24. Sezary syndrome

Wiskott-Aldrich syndrome is characterized by recurrent bacterial infections, hemorrhage secondary to thrombocytopenia and persistant dermatitis. Symptoms including petechiae and ecchymoses occurring on the skin and oral mucosa and signs of hemorrhage on other mucosal surfaces such as epistaxis and hematuria may be observed starting from infancy. Atopic dermatitis-like rash is seen on the face, scalp, ears and the intertriginous areas. Excoriation, thick crusts and lichenification occur due to severe pruritus (Fig. 12.23). External otitis and otitis media are among the common bacterial infections seen in these patients. Systemic infections, hemorrhage and malignancies may lead to death at an early age. In Sezary syndrome and other erythrodermas, intense scaling may occur on the ears (Fig. 12.24). The underlying causes of erythrodermas can be uncovered.

Extramammary Paget's disease is a form of epithelial adenocarcinoma occuring on apocrine-bearing areas of the body such as intertriginous areas and genitalia. The typical lesion is a non-healing, non-pruritic eczematous patch or plaque which may rarely be seen on the external auditory canal.

13 ■ Hyperkeratotic Lesions

The leading cause of ear hyperkeratosis is the genetically inherited disorders of keratinization. It is relatively more prominent on the helix region. In Darier's disease, which usually causes yellow-coloured hyperkeratotic papules mostly in seborrheic areas, involvement of the ears as well as the face and scalp is common. There may be hyperkeratotic lesions on the external ear (Figs. 13.1-13.4). In some patients, coalescent papules may result in hypertrophic plaques, especially on the retroauricular area. An unpleasant odour may occur due to secondary bacterial infections. Although lesions rapidly regress with oral retinoid treatment, recurrence mostly occurs after drug discontinuation. In the KID syndrome, an intense hyperkeratosis may occur on the ear as well as on the tip of the nose (Fig. 13.5). Epidermolytic hyperkeratosis, a severe form of ichthyosis, may cause hyperkeratosis on the ears. Ear hyperkeratosis may accompany certain palmoplantar keratoderma syndromes (Fig. 13.6). Olmsted syndrome leads to severe hyperkeratosis on the palms and soles, periorificial areas and sometimes on the ears. Alopecia and nail dystrophy are other signs of this disease.

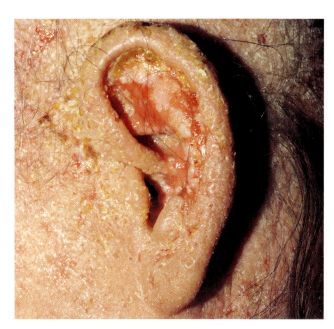

Fig. 13.2. Darier's disease

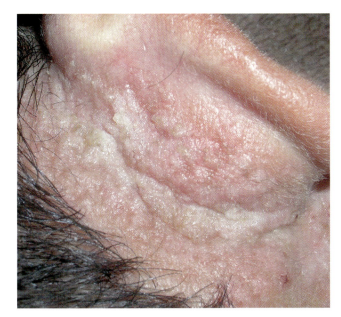

Fig. 13.1. Darier's disease

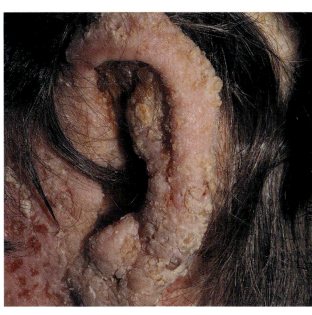

Fig. 13.3. Darier's disease

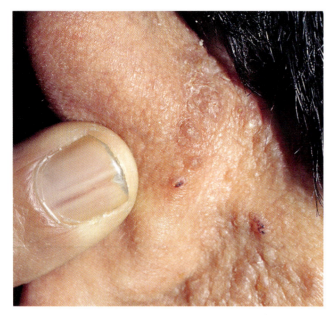

Fig. 13.4. Darier's disease

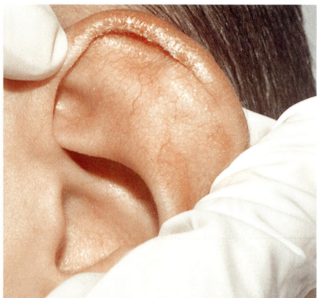

Fig. 13.6. Ear hyperkeratosis accompanying to palmoplantar keratoderma

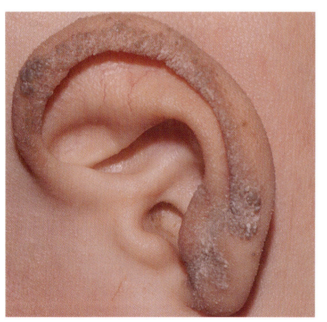

Fig. 13.5. KID syndrmoe

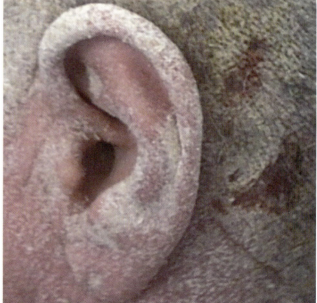

Fig. 13.7. Norwegian scabies

The cardiofacio-cutaneous syndrome is characterized by cardiac abnormalities, developmental delay, downslanting palpebral fissures, peculiar facial appearance including nose deformity, curly sparse hair and skin findings. Keratosis pilaris, palmoplantar keratoderma and hyperkeratotic patches of the ear helix may be seen in this disease.

Scabies is a pruritic disease mostly involving the body and the extremities. A specific form of this infestation, called Norwegian scabies (crusted scabies) is observed mostly in mentally retarded or immunocompromised patients. A very high number of parasites (*Sarcoptes scabiei*) are present in these patients, and lesions may also involve the face and the scalp. The intense hyperkeratotic and scaly lesions of the ears are typical for this form (Fig. 13.7). In contrast to classical scabies, itching may not be severe. On the other hand, the contagiousity of crusted scabies is very high. The causative parasite can be easily detected by scraping material obtained from the lesions. There is no tendency for spontaneous healing, but lesions rapidly disappear following anti-scabies treatment.

Actinic keratosis manifesting as hyperkeratotic, flat or slightly elevated patches with rough surface is common in individuals over middle age with a light skin colour,

13 Hyperkeratotic Lesions

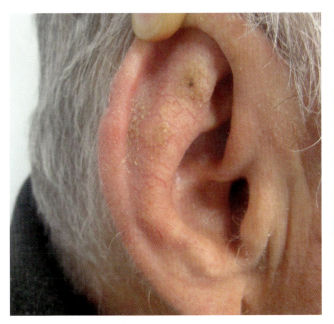

Fig. 13.8. Actinic keratosis

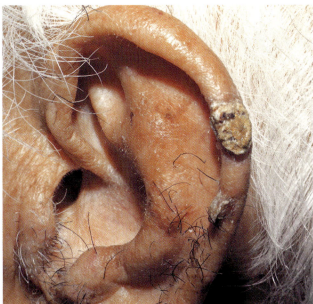

Fig. 13.10. Cutaneous horn

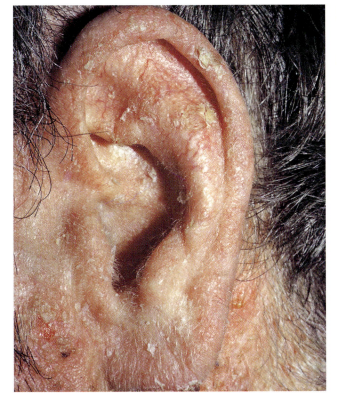

Fig. 13.9. Actinic keratosis

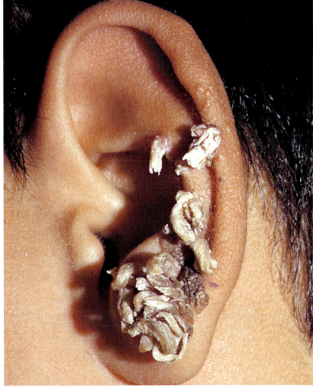

Fig. 13.11. Cutaneous horn on filiform verrucae

who are exposed to intense ultraviolet light cumulatively (Figs. 13.8, 13.9). Some patients may present with multiple lesions on the face, scalp and ears preferentially located on the upper part of the helix. In the hypertrophic form of this in situ carcinoma, lesions are more elevated. Some lesions may be hyperpigmented. As actinic keratosis may trans-form into invasive squamous cell carcinoma, it should be treated. Cutaneous horn may develop secondary to various ear lesions such as filiform verruca, actinic keratosis, keratoacanthoma and squamous cell carcinoma in the form of horn-like extensions (Figs. 13.10-13.12). Therefore, biopsy may be required for the diagnosis of the underlying lesions.

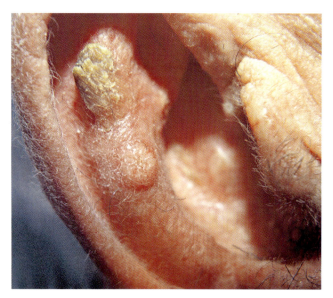 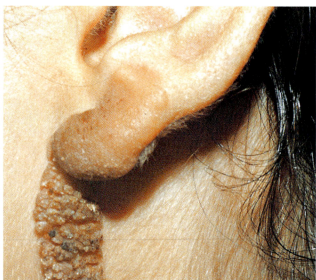

Fig. 13.12. Cutaneous horn on actinic keratosis

Fig. 13.13. Epidermal nevus

Hyperkeratosis may sometimes be striking on the surface of seborrheic keratosis.

When linearly arranged hyperkeratotic papules on a single ear extending to the neck or scalp are seen, epidermal nevus should be considered (Fig. 13.13). This hamartomatous tumor is mostly present after birth. Hyperkeratosis which is mild in infancy becomes severe as the patients get older. Some lesions may have a dark colour. It does not lead to subjective complaints but is a significant cosmetic problem. Diffuse lesions may be part of epidermal nevus syndrome associated with visceral involvement. Following surgical treatment of epidermal nevus, undesirable scars may occur, and there may be recurrence. Elephantiasis nostras verrucosa is characterized by cobblestoned papules and diffuse hyperkeratosis secondary to chronic obstructive lymphedema. It is typically located on the lower extremities, but may also involve the ears. Usually a single ear is affected. Most patients have history of previous attacks of recurrent cellulitis. All other reasons causing lymphedema should be investigated if the history of this streptococcal infection is not present.

In acrokeratosis paraneoplastica (Bazex syndrome), which may potentially accompany squamous cell carcinomas of the upper respiratory tract and the upper gastrointestinal tract, purplish, hyperkeratotic or psoriasis-like plaques may occur on the helix of the ear as well as on the nose and acral parts of the limbs. Cutaneous lesions mostly regress after the treatment of the underlying malignancy.

14 ■ Papular Lesions

Papules due to benign tumors, cutaneous infections, storage disorders and dermatoses triggered by physical or environmental factors are commonly observed on the ear. A few of these disorders are specific to the ear and this has been reflected on the name of these diseases. The ear contains hair follicles, eccrine sweat glands and also some apocrine sweat glands. Therefore, the inflammatory diseases and tumors of the skin appendages may also be seen on the ear.

The open and closed comedones of acne vulgaris may locate particularly on the concha of the ear and may occasionally be huge in size (Fig. 14.1). Comedones may also be observed on the helix, tragus and earlobes. In people with intense solar damage solar elastosis and senile comedones may coexist on the ear (Fig. 14.2). In chloracne which develops after exposure to halogenated aromatic hydrocarbons, large open comedones and yellow cysts may intensely occur on the retroauricular area besides the malar region. These lesions may heal with scars. Molluscum contagiosum may present with bright papules with an umbilicated center on the ears like anywhere else on the body. Typical umbilicated papules and nodules of cryptococcosis, a deep mycosis, may also be located on the ears as well as the nose.

Chondrodermatitis nodularis helicis is a benign condition specific to the ear seen in adults (Figs. 14.3, 14.4). Although not well-established, pressure, actinic damage and cold are thought to be causes of this condition. It most commonly occurs on the preferred sleeping side and is more common on the right ear. It may possibly start after a local cartilage damage which is followed by secondary cutaneous involvement. Helix involvement is more common in men, whereas antihelix involvement in women. Involvement of the upper part of the helix is typical. It may be solitary or may appear as a few

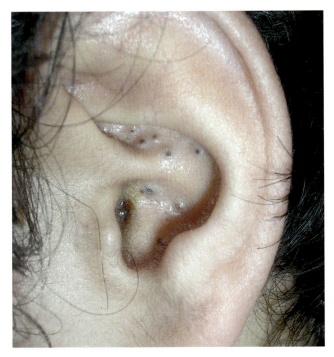

Fig. 14.1. Acne vulgaris. Comedones

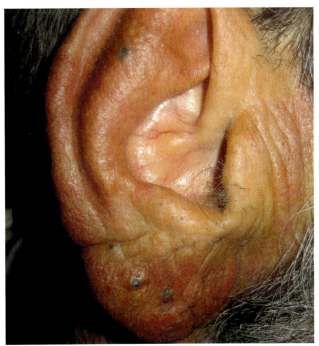

Fig. 14.2. Solar elastosis and senile comedones

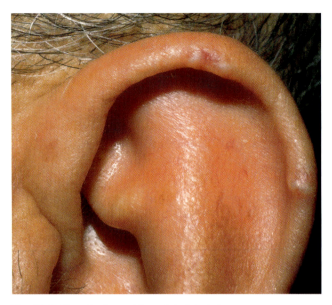

Fig. 14.3. Chondrodermatitis nodularis helicis

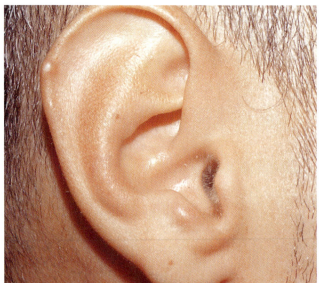

Fig. 14.5. Weathering ear nodules

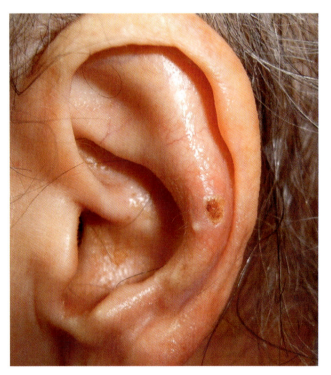

Fig. 14.4. Chondrodermatitis nodularis helicis

lesions featuring as 3 to 8 mm dome-shaped, flesh-coloured, round or oval, firm, painful papules or nodules surrounded by a grey or erythematous rim. Papules are tightly adhered to the cartilage underneath and may have a hyperkeratotic, crusted, eroded or ulcerated surface. The lesions may deteriorate by lying on the same site all the time especially on hard pillows or by using headphones. Pain triggered by pressure may cause sleep disturbance. It may easily be identified by its typical clinical appearance; however biopsy should be obtained in case there is a suspicion of any malignancy. Histopathological changes involve both the skin and the cartilage in chondrodermatitis nodularis helicis. A pressure-relieving cushion may sometimes be helpful but surgical treatment is usually required. Unless the damaged cartilage area is completely excised, recurrence is common. Weathering ear nodules are 2 to 3 mm sized, white- or flesh-coloured firm papules covered with intact skin, which are mostly observed on the free edge of the helix of elderly males with a dense solar damage (Fig. 14.5). Although the lesions are generally small, the term nodule is also included in the title of this disease as in chondrodermatitis nodularis helicis. Inflammation is not observed during the course of the disease. These papules cause no subjective symptoms, but pose a cosmetic problem, especially when bilateral involvement with many lesions develops. In some patients, co-occurrence of weathering ear nodules and chondrodermatitis nodularis helicis is observed. Elastotic nodules of the ear appear as slightly sensitive, waxy papules and nodules adherent to their base which are usually found on the antihelix and rarely on the helix. They do not affect the underlying cartilage. These lesions may be bilateral and sometimes multiple. The signs of chronic solar damage are usually present.

In the late period of the gout which is a purine nucleotide metabolism disorder, the dermal or subcutaneous papules and nodules with size ranging between pinhead or pea are located on the ear, particularly on the helix. These lesions containing monosodium urate crystals are called tophus (Figs. 14.6, 14.7). They are firm, yellowish or cream-coloured and may be painful. Along with ulceration on the surface, white, powder-like contents may discharge over time, however they may recur again. Tophus may also be located on the extremities or sometimes on other regions. Mostly occurring above 40 years

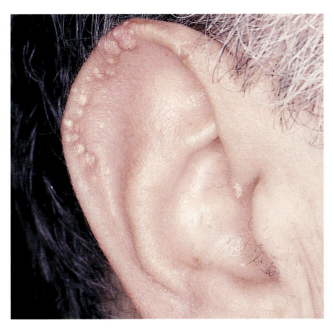

Fig. 14.6. Gout. Tophus

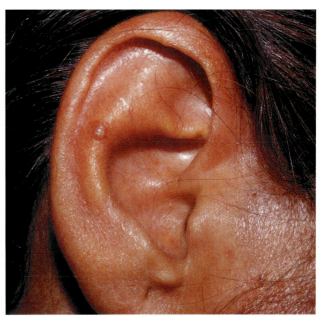

Fig. 14.8. CREST syndrome. Calcinosis cutis

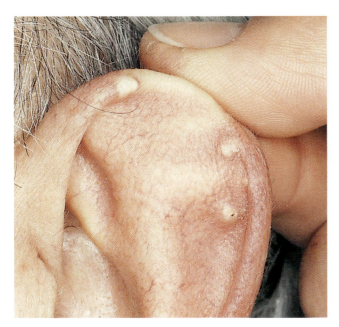

Fig. 14.7. Gout. Tophus

of age, fever, acute and chronic arthritis are the main systemic symptoms of gout. Serum uric acid level is usually elevated. Foods and drugs with a potential to exacerbate gout should be restricted. Therapies aiming to suppress the acute attacks and lower the uric acid level may also be administered. Lesch-Nyhan syndrome manifests with symptoms such as hyperuricemia, mental retardation, spastic cerebral palsy, and tophus-like papules leading to cartilage damage on the auricle. Xanthomas seen in hyperlipidemic patients may rarely occur on the ears as yellow papules and nodules.

White, firm, painless papules on the ears may be noticed in calcinosis cutis. Dystrophic calcification is a type of calcinosis cutis which occurs in patients with localized tissue damage. Connective tissue disorders, particularly CREST syndrome (Fig. 14.8) and juvenile dermatomyositis, are the common and best known causes of this type of calcification on the ears. Auricular calcinosis may also occur in the setting of trauma, perniosis, frostbite, Addison's disease and acromegaly, or sometimes it may be idiopathic. Subepidermal calcified nodule (Winer nodule), a type of idiopathic calcinosis cutis, is most commonly observed on the head and neck, particularly on the ears. It mainly appears as a solitary firm, white, yellowish or sometimes erythematous papule or nodule mainly located on the helix. It may be associated with trauma. Although it is usually observed during childhood, it may occur at any age. When it is present at birth, it is also called congenital calcinosis cutis. Sometimes calcified lesions may ulcerate. Osteoma cutis observed in Albright syndrome manifests as firm papulonodular lesions particularly developing on sites exposed to trauma and pressure and may also involve the ear.

The hyperpigmented, pruritic, papular lesions with a tendency to cropping observed in lichen amyloidosis may rarely be located on the ear especially on the concha. Other signs of primary cutaneous amyloidosis may coexist especially on shins and interscapular area. The disease does not show systemic involvement but has a chronic course. The papulonodular lesions of the primary systemic amyloidosis may particularly appear on the concha of the ear.

In lipoid proteinosis, yellowish tiny papules containing hyaline substance involve the eyelids, ears and other parts of the face. They show tendency to coalesce and typically coexist with cribriform atrophic scars (Fig. 14.9). Hoarseness of the voice from birth is typical in this genodermatosis. Small papules that tend to be grouped on the helix are the typical features of juvenile hyaline fibromatosis, a genodermatosis with progressive fibromatous lesions (Fig. 14.10). Additionally, tumoral masses may be observed on the scalp. Infantile systemic hyalin fibromatosis is characterized by diffuse hyalin deposits in the skin, gastrointestinal tract, muscles and glands. Dermatological manifestations include thickened skin and pearly papules appearing on the neck, face and ears in addition to perianal area. It is usually fatal at the age of 2 years. Juvenile colloid milium manifests with small translucent papules that are frequently located on the ears as well as the face (Figs. 14.11, 14.12).

In scleromyxedema, flesh-coloured, waxy lichenoid papular lesions due to mucin accumulation in the dermis have a tendency to increase in a short time and may be grouped on the retroauricular area (Figs. 14.13, 14.14). The ear may be hardened due to diffuse infiltration. Response to

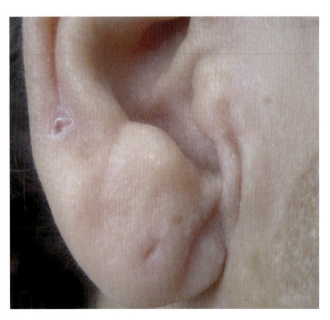

Fig. 14.9. Lipoid proteinosis

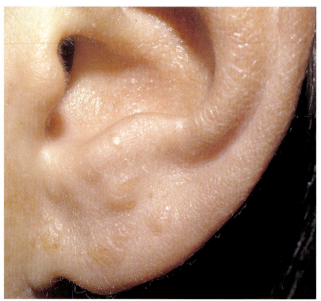

Fig. 14.11. Juvenile colloid milium

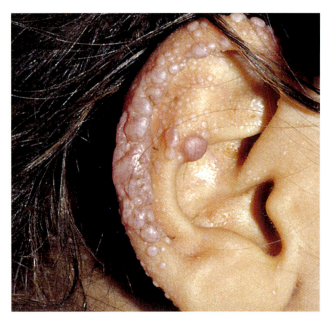

Fig. 14.10. Juvenile hyaline fibromatosis

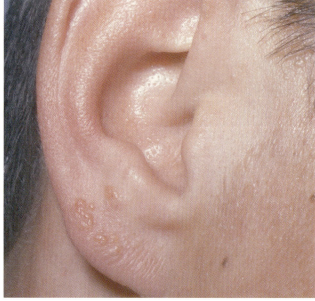

Fig. 14.12. Juvenile colloid milium

treatment is limited in this form of cutaneous mucinosis. Thyroid dermatopathy mainly observed in Graves disease on the pretibial area may also occur on different areas including the earlobes in form of papular lesions.

Eccrine hydrocystoma, though not as common as on the face may manifest as 1 to 3 mm sized, translucent, bluish papules on the ears. Trichilemmomas observed on the ear in Cowden syndrome are flesh- or yellow-coloured, tiny and scattered papules (Figs. 14.15, 14.16). Occasionally, these papules may occupy a considerable part of the pinna. This disease may also cause other mucocutaneous lesions including a cobblestone appearance secondary to papillomas in the mouth, acral keratotic papules on the dorsum of the hands, palmoplantar punctate keratoses, lipomas and hemangiomas. Patients have increased risk of gastrointestinal polyps, soft tissue hamartomas, goitre, breast and thyroid cancer. Fibrofolliculoma or trichodiscomas appear as small, flesh- or greyish yellow-coloured, dome-shaped papules and may be located on the ears. It may be associated with Birt-Hogg-Dubé syndrome (Fig. 14.17) which occurs in young adults leading to disseminated papules on the other parts of the face, neck and trunk. In Brooke-Spiegler syndrome, many trichoepitheliomas consisting of flesh-coloured,

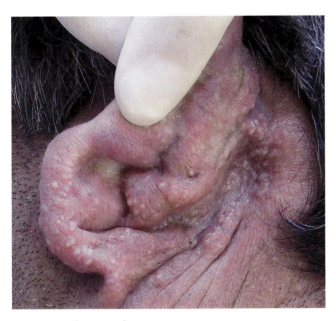

Fig. 14.13. Scleromyxedema

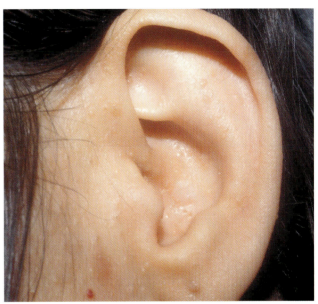

Fig. 14.15. Cowden syndrome. Trichilemmoma

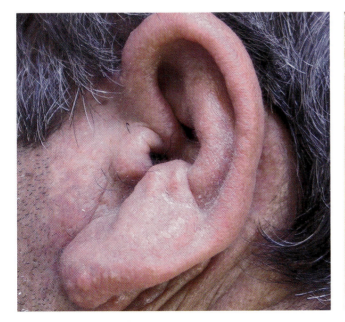

Fig. 14.14. Scleromyxedema

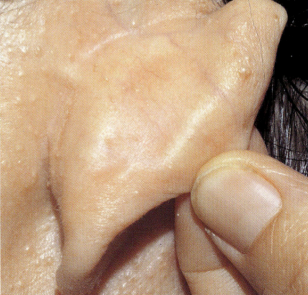

Fig. 14.16. Cowden syndrome. Trichilemmoma

dome-shaped papules and nodules may also be located on the ears besides midface (Fig. 14.18). These lesions have a tendency to be grouped. Papular lesions of angiofibroma related to tuberous sclerosis, mainly involve different parts of the face, but may also be seen on the pinna (Fig. 14.19).

Perniosis (chilblains), a disease developing after long-term exposure to cold below freezing point, involves acral parts such as the fingers, toes, ears and sometimes the nose (Fig. 14.20). In some of these regions, there may be papules and plaques in foci on poorly-demarcated, bluish red or purplish erythematous base. The ears of the patients may be cold and edematous. These lesions may be painful. The disease has quite a chronic course and may deteriorate in the winter. Cryofibrinogenemia is a disease associated with the increase of plasma fibrinogen

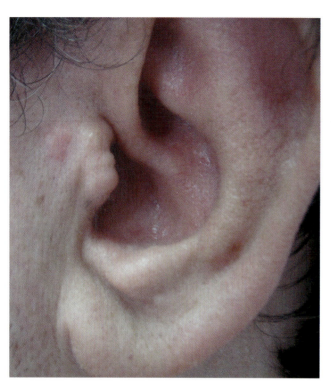

Fig. 14.17. Birt-Hogg-Dubé syndrome. Fibrofolliculoma

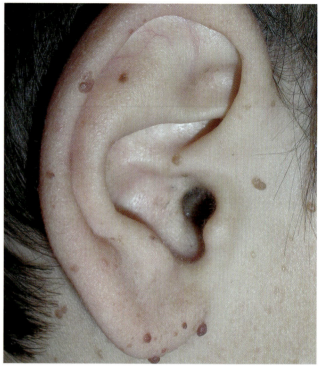

Fig. 14.19. Tuberous sclerosis

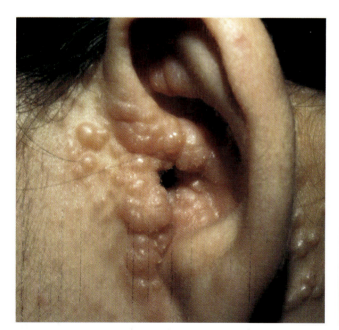

Fig. 14.18. Trichoepithelioma

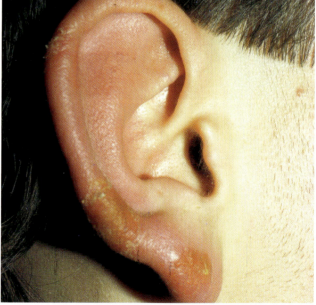

Fig. 14.20. Perniosis

which typically precipitates in cold and leads to ulceration, hemorrhage and purpura especially on acral regions such as the extremities, nose and ears (Fig. 14.21). It is usually associated with malignancies, thromboembolic diseases, diabetes mellitus or medication. In secondary syphilis, copper-red papular lesions may occasionally develop on the ear. The diagnosis is usually established by the presence of other lesions in typical regions and confirmed by serological tests.

Polymorphic light eruption is a chronic disease characterized by attacks that occur hours or days after exposure to ultraviolet light (Fig. 14.22). Its' onset is usually in spring or early summer. Itchy, erythematous papules on the forearms, dorsum of the hands, legs, decolette, face and also ears are the typical features. Other lesions such as plaques, urticarial lesions, vesicles and eczematous lesions can also be seen. Although the attacks settle in 7 to 10 days, new lesions may occur if complete sun protection is not achieved. In actinic reticuloid, a disease associated with chronic ultraviolet light damage, diffuse infiltration may occur on the ears as well as the face. The monomorphous eruption of 1 to 3 mm sized papules in lupus miliaris

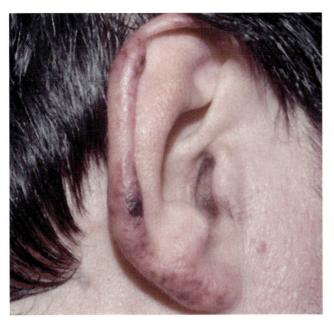

Fig. 14.21. Cryofibrinogenemia

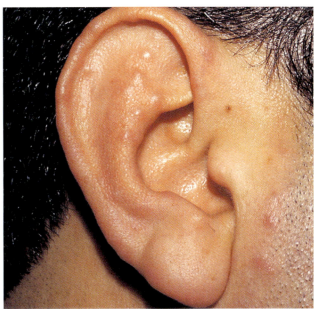

Fig. 14.23. Lupus miliaris disseminatus faciei

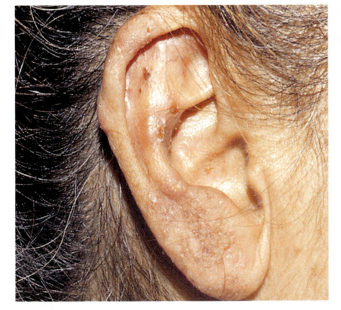

Fig. 14.22. Polymorphic light eruption

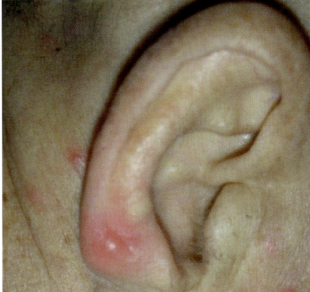

Fig. 14.24. Insect bite

disseminatus faciei locates mainly on the midface, however, papules may also be observed on the ears (Fig. 14.23).

Elastosis perforans serpiginosa results from extrusion of the degenerated elastic fibers of the dermis through epidermis and is characterized by 2 to 5 mm sized horny papules arranged in a linear or annular form. These lesions are particularly located on the neck and limbs but may occasionaly be observed on the ears unilaterally. They may be idiopathic or develop in association with other connective tissue disorders and Down's syndrome or may be associated with D-penicillamine use. Reticulate atrophic scars occur after regression of these lesions.

In cyclosporine-induced folliculodystrophy, which is a rare drug reaction, flesh-coloured follicular papules may be so intense that they cover the entire external ear. Insect bites occur frequently on the ear, a region susceptible to external factors (Fig. 14.24). This cutaneous reaction caused by biting or stinging of arthropods presents typically as itchy erythematous and edematous papules. Some lesions have an intact vesicle or crust at the center. The number of the lesions is variable, and typically facial lesions coexist. They regress after a short time without treatment.

15 ■ Nodular Lesions

The main causes of the nodular lesions observed on the ears are benign or malignant tumors. Additionally, some congenital abnormalities, infections and inflammatory dermatoses may also cause nodules on the ears. Especially, large nodules on the ears may be disfiguring.

Congenital melanocytic nevi may be seen on the ears like anywhere else on the body (Fig. 15.1). Congenital giant hairy nevi of the scalp and neck may also involve the ears (Fig. 15.2). As the excision of these nevi may result in tissue loss causing prominent cosmetic problems, it is difficult to decide about a prophylactic excision of the ear lesions. All types of common acquired melanocytic nevi can be seen on the ears and they can generally be diagnosed clinically. Junctional nevi mostly occur in childhood as brown-coloured, 2 to 5 mm sized, flat or slightly raised lesions (Fig. 15.3). They are not true nodules but are mentioned here because of their differential diagnostic importance in the spectrum of melanocytic nevi. Although rare when compared to other areas of the face, intradermal nevi may also be seen on the ears

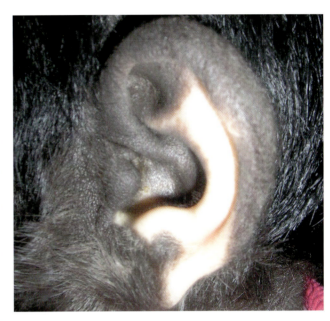

Fig. 15.2. Congenital giant hairy nevus

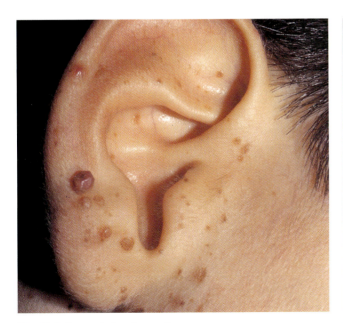

Fig. 15.1. Congenital melanocytic nevus

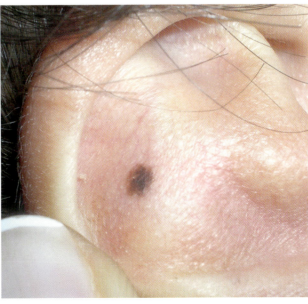

Fig. 15.3. Junctional nevus

especially in middle-aged women (Fig. 15.4). These flesh- or light brown-coloured, elevated, soft papules or nodules with well-defined borders may have a few hairs projecting from the surface. Compound nevus may have two components, one of them being more elevated than the other (Fig. 15.5). Some compound and intradermal nevi have papillomatous surface (Fig. 15.6). There is no indication to remove the acquired melanocytic nevi which do not show any atypical changes. The typical dome-shaped papules or nodules of Spitz nevus varying from pink to dark brown in colour may be located on the ears (Fig. 15.7). On the other hand, blue nevus presenting as a grey-, black- or blue-coloured, regular, round or oval papule or nodule with a smooth surface is rarely seen on the ears (Fig. 15.8). This type of nevus is usually solitary. Multiple blue nevi may be associated with LAMB syndrome (Carney complex). Spitz nevus and blue nevus are benign tumors with a very low chance of malignant degeneration. Therefore, routine excision is not indicated for these nevi. However, if there are any diagnostic difficulties, histologic evaluation is mandatory.

Malignant melanoma is the leading cause of death from skin disease, and approximately 1-4% of these tumors are

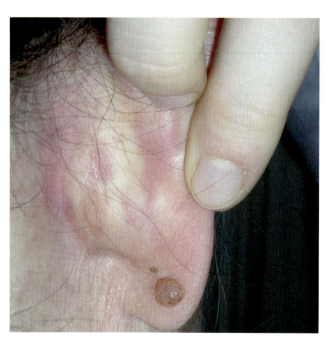

Fig. 15.4. Intradermal nevus

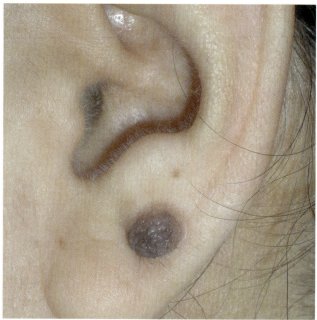

Fig. 15.6. Compound nevus. Papillomatous nevus

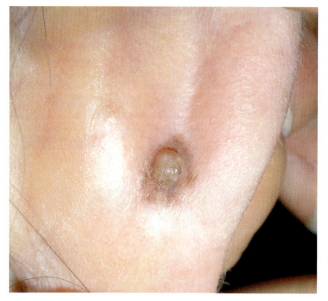

Fig. 15.5. Compound nevus

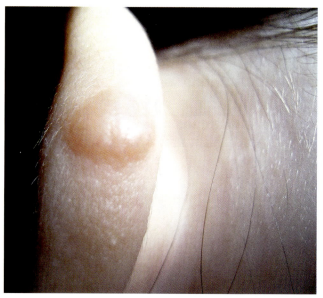

Fig. 15.7. Spitz nevus

located on the ears. Various types of malignant melanoma may be seen on this region. Lentigo malignant melanoma especially involves helix and antihelix, the ear parts that are more exposed to ultraviolet light (Fig. 15.9). This type of malignant melanoma has a relatively good prognosis but if neglected, papules and nodules occur on irregular pigmented macules over time indicating the invasive stage of the disease (Fig. 15.10). Surface ulceration is frequently present on the nodular component of the tumors, and its presence significantly worsens the prognosis. The initial lesion of nodular malignant melanoma is a brown or black papule that changes to a nodule within months or years. It may also be located on the ears (Fig. 15.11) and may occasionally originate from the external auditory canal. Desmoplastic malignant melanoma with relatively light-coloured nodules and amelanotic malignant melanoma with depigmented or sometimes ulcerated nodules may also be seen on the ears. Surgical procedures need to be performed with wide margins, especially for nodules in the invasive stage of malignant melanoma. Therefore, it poses great cosmetic problems in this area. Satellites of primary malignant melanoma and cutaneous metastatic malignant melanoma may manifest as multiple pigmented

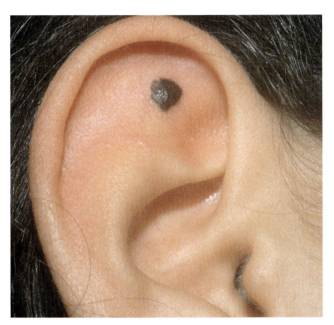

Fig. 15.8. Blue nevus

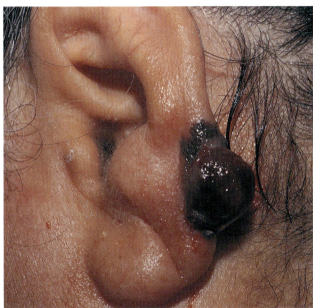

Fig. 15.10. Lentigo malignant melanoma (late stage)

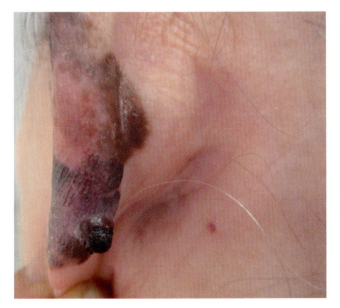

Fig. 15.9. Lentigo malignant melanoma (late stage)

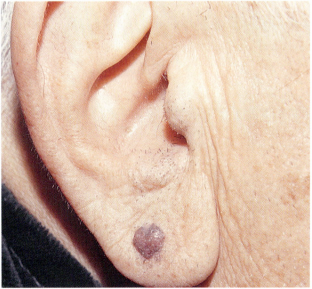

Fig. 15.11. Nodular malignant melanoma

papules and nodules on the ears (Fig. 15.12). Furthermore, malignant blue nevus may also occur on the ears. This tumor tends to show progressive enlargement and may be associated with intracranial involvement. Regional lymph nodes are the common sites of metastasis. Pigmented basal cell carcinoma is another tumor which should be remembered in the differential diagnosis of the pigmented nodules in this area. A histopathological examination is usually necessary for definitive diagnosis.

Epidermoid cyst primarily involves antihelix and earlobe as a dome-shaped, smooth-surfaced, mobile nodule (Fig. 15.13). On the other hand, multiple epidermoid cysts and milia may sometimes be encountered on the retroauricular area. Milia an

plaque, a rare lesion which presents as multiple milia on an erythematous base is frequently seen on and around the ears.

Acne vulgaris cysts can be palpated as deep swellings and can also be located on the retroauricular region (Fig. 15.14). These lesions are mostly associated with comedones.

Auricular pseudocyst is a nodular ear lesion with a smooth surface which does not have a true cyst wall (Fig. 15.15). Chronic trauma has been suggested in the etiology. It is usually seen unilaterally on the helix and antihelix, especially in the scaphoid fossa of middle-aged men. It is a firm, painless swelling with intact surface that contains a clear fluid with glycosaminoglycans. It slowly enlarges in 2 to 3 months, reaches 1-5 cm in diameter, and may be fluctuating. Treatment options

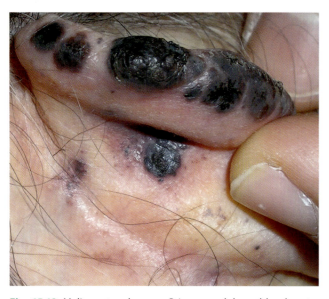

Fig. 15.12. Malignant melanoma. Primary nodule and local metastatic lesions

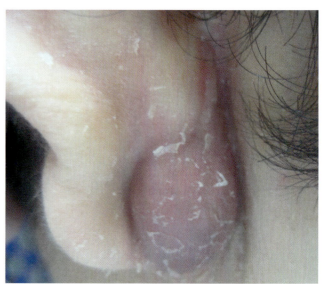

Fig. 15.14. Acne vulgaris. Cyst

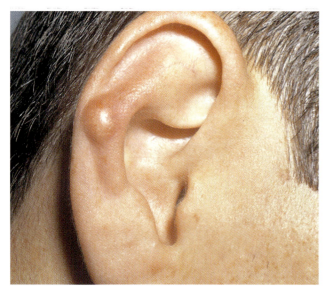

Fig. 15.13. Epidermoid cyst

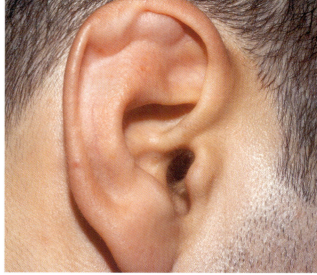

Fig. 15.15. Auricular pseudocyst

such as aspiration, drainage or intralesional injection of corticosteroids have the risk of development of perichondritis (inflammation of the cartilage and the surrounding vascular structures) and deformity. The aspiration fluid material is yellow or orange in colour, and in olive-oil consistency.

Preauricular sinus is a congenital defect that seems like a cystic nodule or an opening (Fig. 15.16). The incidence changes between 0.1-10% in different countries, and there may be a positive family history. It develops as a result of imperfect embryologic fusion of the primitive ear tubercles. It is located on the preauricular area (in the front or anterior crux of the helix), usually being unilateral and right-sided. It may be a small superficial pit or a deep sinus and is located outside the temporal facia without involving the tympanic membrane or external auditory canal. The sinus very occasionally tracks deeply to the facial nerve. If the epithelia of the sinuses become infected, erythema, tenderness and purulent discharge with unpleasant odour can be observed (Fig. 15.17). Most patients are otherwise healthy. Preauricular sinuses may sometimes be associated with hearing loss and renal abnormalities as in cases with branchio-oto-renal syndrome and also may be seen in a number of other congenital conditions such as Treacher-Collins syndrome, Waardenburg syndrome and trisomy 22 mosaicism. Renal ultrasound examination and auditory testing should be performed in cases with other congenital abnormalities. While complete excision is definitely indicated in the recurrent infected preauricular sinuses, some authors also recommend excision of the asymptomatic ones.

Neurofibroma is a benign nerve sheath tumor which may locate on the ear like anywhere else on the body (Figs. 15.18-15.20). Soft, flaccid, flesh-coloured nodules 0.2 to 2 cm in diameter are usually asymptomatic. However, some neurofibromas may be destructive via spreading the cranial nerves. Lipoma, a benign tumor composed of fat tissue, may occasionally locate on the ears of adults as soft, flesh-coloured subcutaneous swellings. Angiolipoleiomyoma (angiomyolipoma) is a benign tumor of the kidneys which may rarely be encountered on the skin. It may involve the nose and ears presenting with slowly-growing, painless, firm nodules (Fig. 15.21). Although it has been suggested that tuberous sclerosis must be searched in these patients, an association could not be determined in most cases.

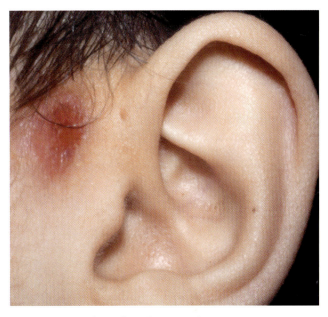

Fig. 15.17. Secondary infected preauricular sinus

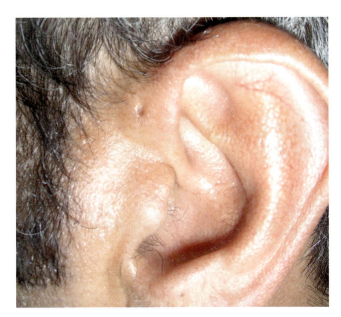

Fig. 15.16. Preauricular sinus

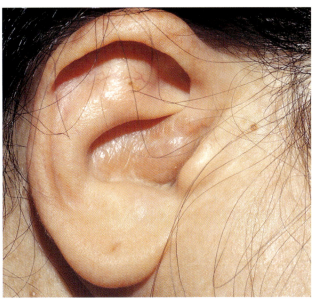

Fig. 15.18. Neurofibroma

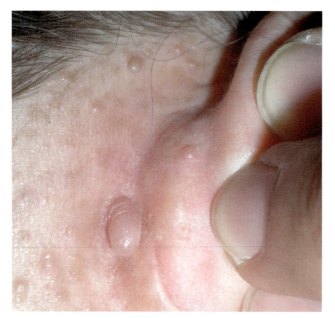

Fig. 15.19. Neurofibroma

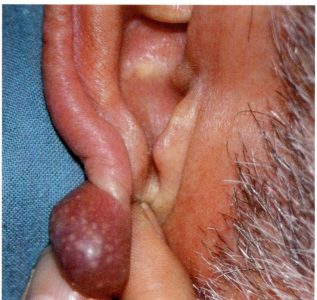

Fig. 15.21. Angiolipoleiomyoma

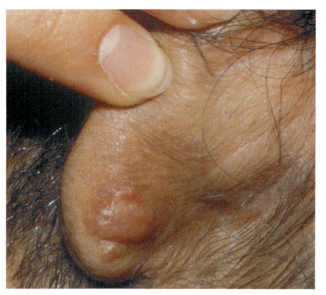

Fig. 15.20. Neurofibroma

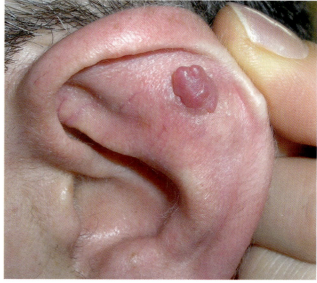

Fig. 15.22. Pilomatricoma

Pilomatricoma is a hair follicle tumor which has a predilection for the head and neck area. Firm, painless, 0.5 to 3 cm sized subcutaneous nodules may be seen on the ears (Fig. 15.22). Most of the cases are children. Cylindroma, a benign tumor of sweat gland origin, may appear sporadically as a solitary nodule or as multiple lesions associated with Brooke-Spiegler syndrome (Figs. 15.23, 15.24). These tumors have a predilection to occur on the scalp and ears. They appear as rubber-like, pinkish, smooth-surfaced nodules with prominent telangiectases. Their size varies from a few millimeters to several centimeters. Some large lesions may even cause disfigurement. In Brooke-Spiegler syndrome, trichoepithelioma, eccrine spiradenoma, milia, basal cell carcinoma and basal cell adenoma of the parotid gland may also be observed. Eccrine spiradenoma is characterized by flesh- or bluish-coloured, firm, large nodules. This painful tumor rarely involves the ears. Apocrine hidrocystoma (cystadenoma) is a benign cystic tumor of the apocrine secretory glands causing dome-shaped, bluish, translucent nodules on the head and neck area including the ears. Chondroid syringoma is another sweat gland tumor which sometimes appears on the ears as flesh-coloured subcutaneous nodules

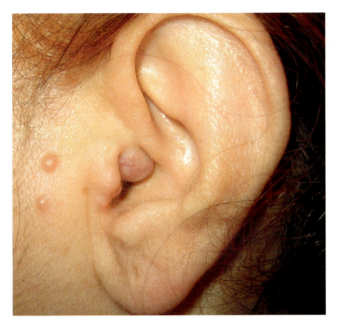

Fig. 15.23. Cylindroma. Brooke-Spiegler syndrome

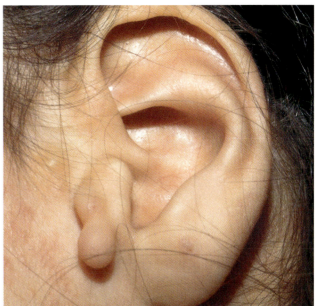

Fig. 15.25. Accessory tragus

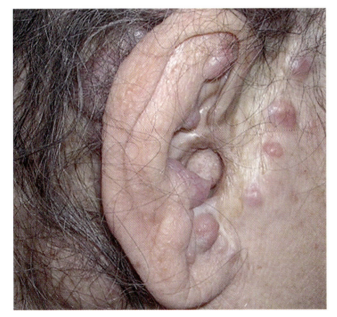

Fig. 15.24. Cylindroma

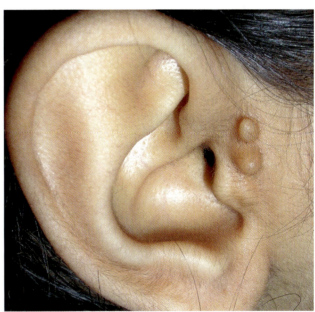

Fig. 15.26. Accessory tragus

and can not easily be diagnosed without histopathological examination.

Accessory tragus is a congenital malformation resulting from the ectopic cartilage rests of the primitive tubercles forming the ear in the embryonic life. It may be observed on the face, on an imaginary line drawn from the tragus to the angle of the mouth or along the anterior margin of the sternocleidomastoid muscle in 0.2-0.5% of the population (Figs. 15.25, 15.26). It is more commonly located on or near tragus as a solitary lesion or a few lesions. A flesh-coloured nodule smaller than 1 cm with smooth surface is typically observed. The nodule may sometimes be pedunculated or lobular. There may be vellus hairs on the surface. Palpation of the lesion reveals either cartilage tissue or skin only. However, the central cartilaginous core is a diagnostic clue. The asymptomatic lesion only poses cosmetic concerns. Rarely, it is associated with congenital syndromes such as Goldenhar syndrome (oculo-auriculo-vertebral syndrome), Naegeli-Franceschetti-Jadassohn syndrome, Nager syndrome,

Treacher-Collins syndrome, Wolf-Hirschhorn syndrome, oculocerebrocutaneous syndrome, Townes-Brocks syndrome and VACTERL association (vertebral abnormalities, anal atresia, cardiac malformation, tracheoesophagieal fistula, renal abnormalities, extremity abnormalities). As accessory tragus does not lead to any complications, it can be left untreated. The decision to excise for cosmetic reasons should be made bearing in mind that the ectopic cartilage tissue could be deep, therefore cauterization should be avoided. The Cri du chat syndrome (deletion 5p syndrome) is a genetic disease associated with various sized deletions of the short arm of chromosome 5. High-pitched, cat-like cry is a characteristic clinical feature. The other main clinical features are microcephaly, broad nasal bridge, epicanthal folds, micrognathia, abnormal dermatoglyphics, prematurely grey hair, ear deformities, severe motor and mental retardation. Additionally, preauricular tags can be seen which may be confused with accessory tragus. Syndactyly, hypospadias, cryptorchidism, neurological and renal abnormalities are other rare findings of the syndrome. Darwin tubercle is a congenital abnormality which is observed as a small prominence at the posterior superior aspect of the helix and is called as the "elf ear" during childhood (Fig. 15.27). Though it is only a cosmetic problem, it may pose some psychological problems in children, thus excision may be considered. The lesion may sometimes be familial.

Traumatic hematoma of the auricle (hematoma auris) is collection of blood under the auricular perichondrium. It is mostly seen as a result of rough contacts in sports like wrestling, boxing, rugby. Lesions are typically located on the scaphoid fossa and triangular fossa due to the rupture of small vessels. This hematoma is painless and inflamation is minimal. It persists unless drained. In these cases it may result with a cauliflower-like deformity due to fibrosis of cartilage (wrestler's ear). The early diagnosis of the hematoma and appropriate surgical intervention can reduce the cosmetic deformity.

Ceruminoma (hidradenoma of the external auditory canal) is a rare benign tumor originating from apocrine ceruminous glands of the skin lining the cartilaginous part of the external auditory canal. It may present with hard subcutaneous nodules obstructing the ear canal causing unilateral conductive hearing loss. On the other hand, tumors such as adenocarcinoma or adenoid cystic carcinoma may also develop from the ceruminous glands of the ears. As these tumors have tendency for local invasion, early diagnosis and excision may avoid the complications.

The earlobe is one of the common locations of keloid which is a hyperproliferative response of connective tissue to trauma (Figs. 15.28-15.30). Ear piercing is a major cause of the earlobe keloid. Sometimes local infections may also be causative factor. Most of them are located on the back side of the earlobes and may sometimes be bilateral. It may be seen on the other areas of the ears developing secondary to piercing in atypical location. Raised, firm, irregularly shaped, pink or reddish brown nodules and plaques with a smooth, shiny surface may sometimes be itchy. Keloid may also spread beyond the traumatized area. The management of keloid is difficult. Although it may regress following treatment with intralesional corticosteroids, cryotherapy, excision or radiotherapy, recurrences are frequent. Therefore, people with a tendency to develop keloid should be warned against the risk of ear piercing.

Hypertrophic scar is differentiated from keloid by confining to the trauma area (Fig. 15.31). Surgical procedures may cause hypertrophic scar on the ear. Lobomycosis (keloidal blastomycosis) is a rare type of deep mycosis characterized

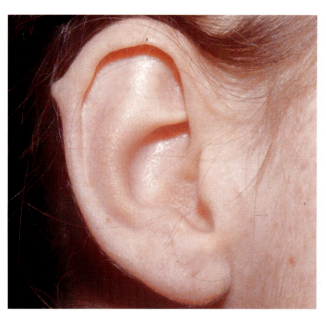

Fig. 15.27. Darwin tubercle

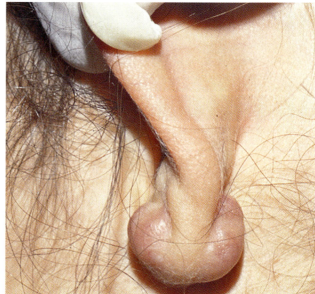

Fig. 15.28. Keloid

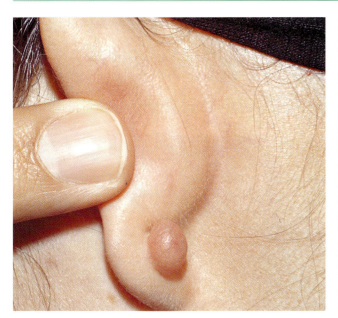

Fig. 15.29. Keloid

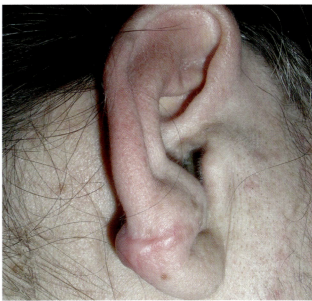

Fig. 15.31. Hypertrophic scar

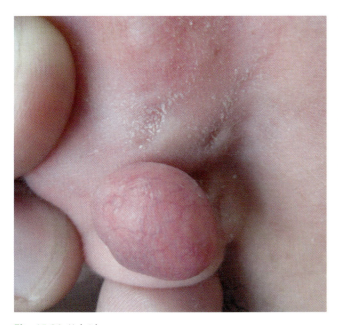

Fig. 15.30. Keloid

with pseudokeloidal nodules with or without fistulas. Ear involvement with multiple violet to pink nodules causing "cauliflower ear" appearance is typical.

Lymphocytoma cutis is a type of pseudolymphoma which may be seen on the ears as reddish brown or reddish purple, firm, persistent nodules with smooth surface. In regions with endemic *Borrelia burgdorferi* infection (Lyme disease) the spirochaete may be the antigenic stimulus inducing the pseudolymphomas, especially located on the earlobe. While ear pseudolymphomas are often idiopathic, it has also been suggested that earrings could trigger pseudolymphomas on the ear. Lymphocytoma cutis resembles cutaneous B cell lymphomas histopathologically. However, it has a benign course. Lymphocytic infiltration of the skin (Jessner-Kanof disease) which is a T cell pseudolymphoma, can be observed as a solitary or a few, asymptomatic erythematous plaques located on the face, chest and rarely on the ears. B cell chronic lymphocytic leukemia can cause nodules or infiltrative plaques resembling pseudolymphoma especially on the earlobe. Cutaneous B cell lymphomas like marginal zone lymphoma rarely involve the ear (Fig. 15.32). Auricle may also be involved in the tumoral stage of mycosis fungoides (Fig. 15.33). These lesions may be ulcerated.

Some types of non-Langerhans cell histiocytosis may cause nodules on the ears. Multicentric reticulohistiocytosis is commonly observed in adults and has a predilection to locate on acral regions. Apart from extremities, it may cause yellow or reddish brown, firm papules or nodules on the ears and nose. Mucosal involvement and severe arthropathy accompany the skin lesions. Malignancies may occur in some patients. Juvenile xanthogranuloma, another non-Langerhans cell histiocytosis, may cause yellowish, solitary or a few papulonodular lesions on the ears (Fig. 15.34, 15.35). The disease is usually idiopathic and localized to the skin. Rarely, it may be associated with chronic myeloid leukemia and neurofibromatosis. The reasonable approach to the ear lesions is to wait for spontaneous regression. The eruption of benign cephalic histiocytosis generally begins during the first three years of life as reddish yellow, slightly raised, 2 to 4 mm sized papules or nodules on the face and ears (Fig. 15.36). Spontaneous regression occurs in a few years, mostly leaving pigmentation. Langerhans cell histiocytosis may cause papules or nodules on the ear as well as eczematous lesions

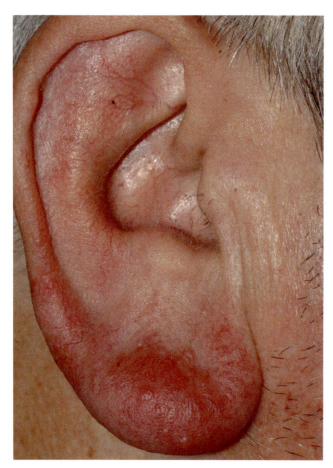

Fig. 15.32. Marginal zone B cell lymphoma

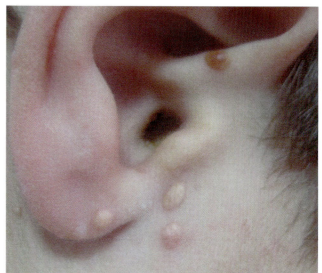

Fig. 15.34. Juvenile xanthogranuloma

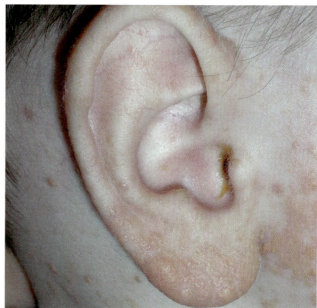

Fig. 15.35. Juvenile xanthogranuloma. Disseminated lesions

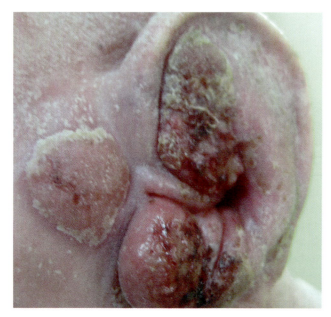

Fig. 15.33. Mycosis fungoides

(Fig. 15.37). Chronic otitis is a common complication of this disease.

All types of basal cell carcinoma may involve the ears (Figs. 15.38, 15.39). The lesions may locate anywhere on the ear including the retroauricular area. Basal cell carcinomas of the concha may infiltrate periosteum and the external auditory canal. Tumors located on the retroauricular area may invade the cartilage. Recurrence is relatively common if ear lesions are not treated with Mohs' microsurgery. Squamous cell carcinoma may locate anywhere

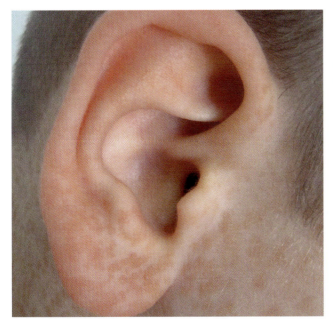

Fig. 15.36. Benign cephalic histiocytosis

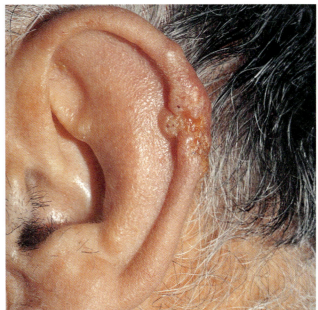

Fig. 15.38. Basal cell carcinoma

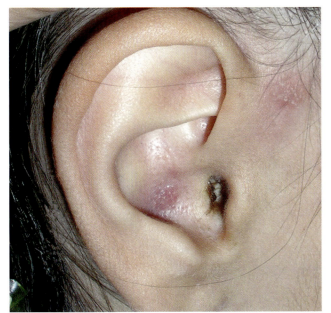

Fig. 15.37. Langerhans cell histiocytosis

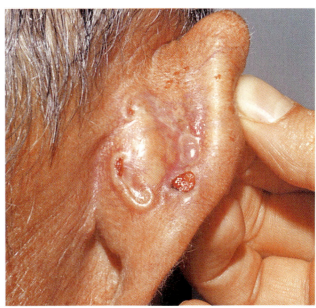

Fig. 15.39. Basal cell carcinoma

on the ear, but more frequently on the helix (Fig. 15.40). It may sometimes develop on a preexisting actinic keratosis. The invasive lesions of the external auditory canal may result in hearing loss and facial nerve paralysis. Bowen's disease on the ear may cause slightly raised plaques, while keratoacanthoma (Fig. 15.41) causes typical punched-out nodules with a crateriform appearance. Atypical fibroxanthoma is a sarcomatous skin tumor seen on sun-exposed areas of elderly and may present with rapidly-growing 1-2 cm sized nodules and plaques on the ear. Some tumors may be ulcerated. Merkel cell carcinoma can also be seen on the ear of elderly as a non-ulcerated solitary nodule mimicking hemangioma. The tumor showing neuroendocrine differentiation frequently causes distant metastasis. Carcinoma of the parotid gland may show invasion to the ear in the late stage (Fig. 15.42).

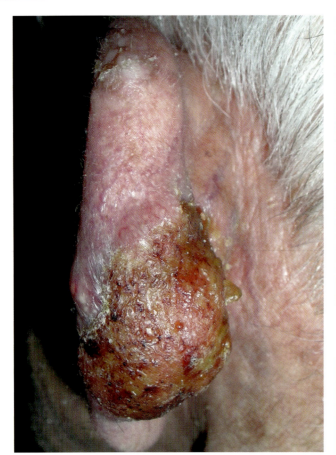

Fig. 15.40. Squamous cell carcinoma

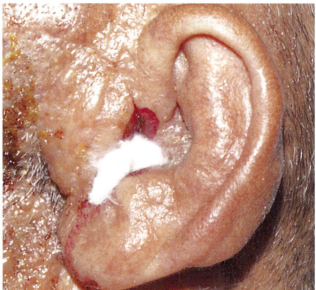

Fig. 15.42. Parotid carcinoma

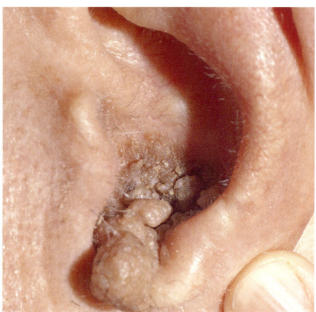

Fig. 15.43. Seborrheic keratosis

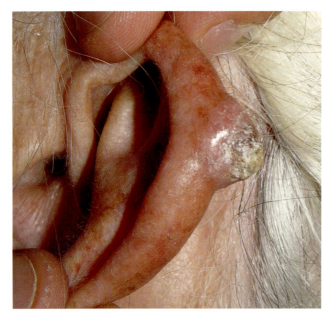

Fig. 15.41. Keratoacanthoma

Seborrheic keratosis is usually seen after middle age as papulonodular lesions in different sizes on any part of the ears (Figs. 15.43-15.47). It may be flat or raised with a rough surface. Tiny, embedded keratin cysts on the surface can be noticed. The colour of the tumor may be yellow, brown or black. Nevus sebaceous is a congenital hamartomatous lesion which occurs mostly on the scalp and face, and sometimes on the ear. Yellow-coloured, tiny papules coalesce to form hairless plaques. They appear in many directions from

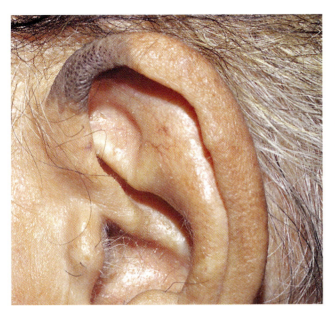

Fig. 15.44. Seborrheic keratosis

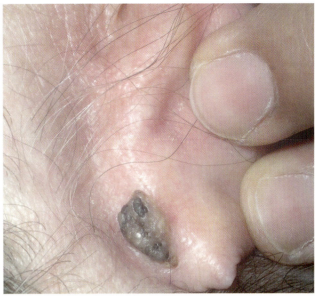

Fig. 15.46. Seborrheic keratosis

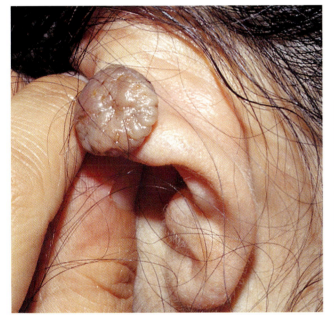

Fig. 15.45. Seborrheic keratosis

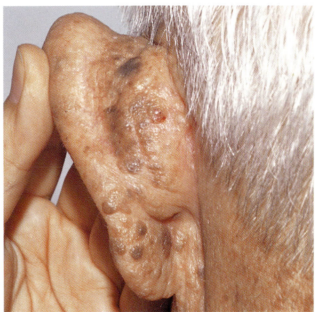

Fig. 15.47. Seborrheic keratosis

the temples to the pinna, from the scalp to the retroauricular area, or only locate on the pinna (Fig. 15.48-15.50). There is a risk of development of other tumors on nevus sebaceous such as trichoblastoma and basal cell carcinoma. However, a consensus for a prophylactic excision has not been established. The decision for excision is difficult when the lesion locates on regions like ears where cosmetic results would not be satisfactory. Isolated mastocytoma may occasionally arise on the ear as a reddish brown, solitary nodule or plaque in early childhood. This lesion usually involutes spontaneously.

Different vascular tumors may cause nodules on the ears. The most typical location for infantile capillary hemangioma is the head and neck, so it can be frequently observed on the ear (Figs. 15.51, 15.52). Ulceration is more commonly seen on the ear lesions (Fig. 15.53). While secondary infection of hemangiomas in these regions can cause destruction of the underlying tissues, large lesions can obstruct the external

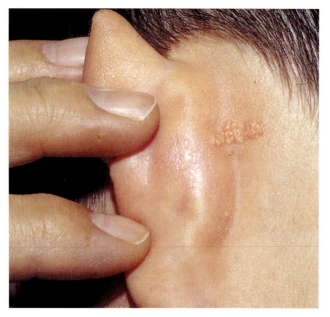

Fig. 15.48. Nevus sebaceous

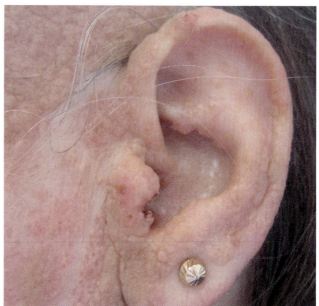

Fig. 15.50. Nevus sebaceous

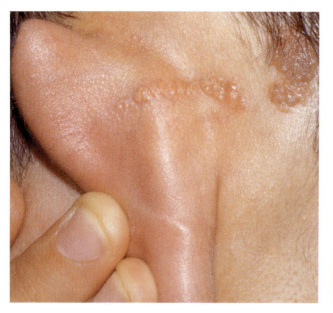

Fig. 15.49. Nevus sebaceous

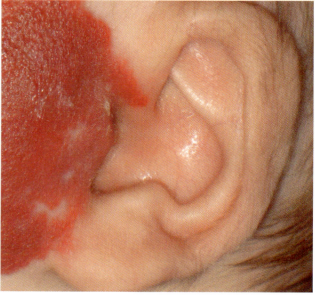

Fig. 15.51. Infantile capillary hemangioma

auditory canal and cause hearing loss (Fig. 15.54). In these cases, systemic treatments such as high dose corticosteroids are indicated to reduce the size of the hemangioma. Arteriovenous malformations may also be located on the ear, usually unilaterally. The entire pinna may be affected with the lateral aspects of the scalp and neck. These lesions may be congenital or may appear later. It presents with asymptomatic macules like nevus flammeus or telangiectases (Fig. 15.55). They develop into pulsatile masses within years (Figs. 15.56, 15.57). Auscultation reveals a thrill-like sound. Necrosis, ulceration and hemorrhage can be life threatening in late stages of arteriovenous malformation which may then require radical surgery.

Benign vascular proliferation and blood eosinophilia are the features of angiolymphoid hyperplasia with eosinophilia which commonly occurs on the ears (Figs. 15.58-15.60). Young adults are usually affected, and 0.5 to 1 cm, red or purple, multiple, grouped papules or subcutaneos nodules are found mostly on the concha and retroauricular area. The surface of these tumors is usually smooth. Erosions,

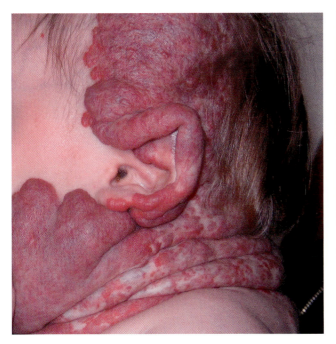
Fig. 15.52. Infantile capillary hemangioma

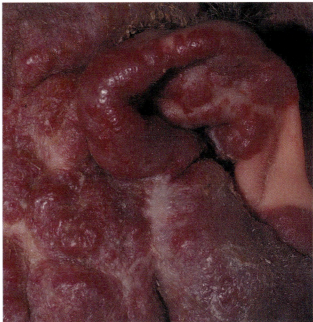
Fig. 15.54. Infantile capillary hemangioma

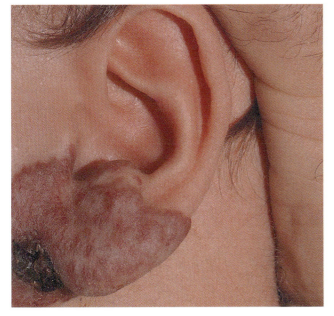
Fig. 15.53. Infantile capillary hemangioma

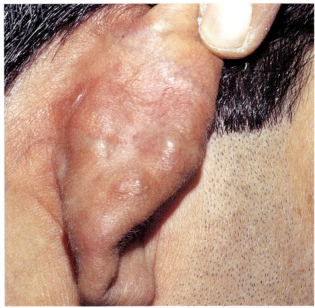
Fig. 15.55. Arteriovenous malformation. Early stage

ulcerations or bleeding occur occasionally. Recurrences are common, despite all possible therapies (Fig. 15.61). Head and neck region is the typical location for Kimura disease characterized by peripheral eosinophilia, lymphadenopathy and vascular tumors. This causes subcutaneous nodules or masses on the preauricular area and parotid gland. Involvement may be bilateral, and renal lesions may accompany the disease. Pyogenic granuloma presents as a red, exophytic nodule with eroded surface on the ears (Fig. 15.62). This tumor grows rapidly at the beginning, but has a tendency for spontaneous resolution. Therefore, aggressive procedures for ear lesions must be avoided. Widespread hemangiomas of blue rubber bleb nevus syndrome may also involve the ears (Fig. 15.63). Hemangiomas in gastrointestinal tract may cause severe complications in this syndrome.

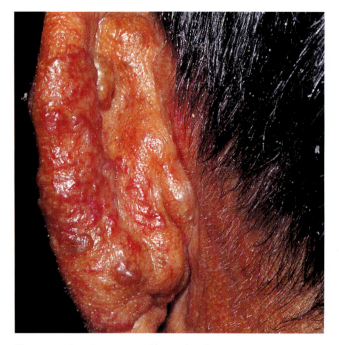

Fig. 15.56. Arteriovenous malformation. Late stage

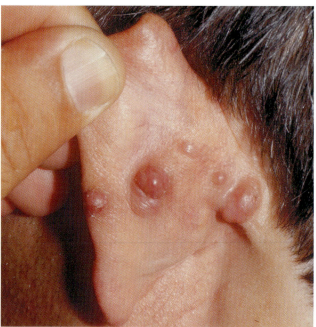

Fig. 15.58. Angiolymphoid hyperplasia with eosinophilia

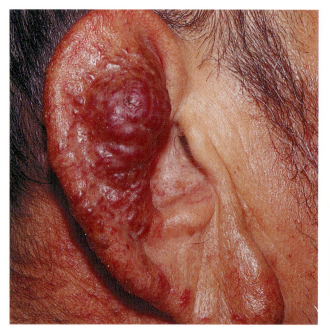

Fig. 15.57. Arteriovenous malformation. Late stage

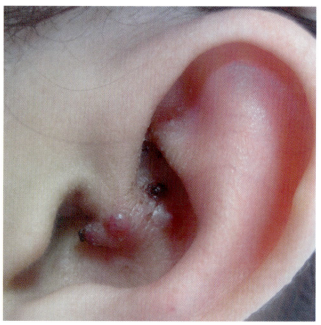

Fig. 15.59. Angiolymphoid hyperplasia with eosinophilia

One of the typical sites of venous lake (phlebectasia) is the ear (Figs. 15.64, 15.65). Lesions may be multiple and involve different parts of the ear. Soft, dark blue swellings are easily compressible. A diagnostic clue is the fading of the lesion on pressure with glass (Fig. 15.66). Even though the lesions are persistent, they do not lead to any complications. Kaposi's sarcoma is another disease presenting with red, brown or purple vascular nodules and plaques on the ears (Figs. 15.67, 15.68). The helix, antihelix, earlobe, retroauricular area and external auditory canal may be involved. Kaposi's sarcoma associated with HIV infection involves the ear more commonly. The size of the nodules is

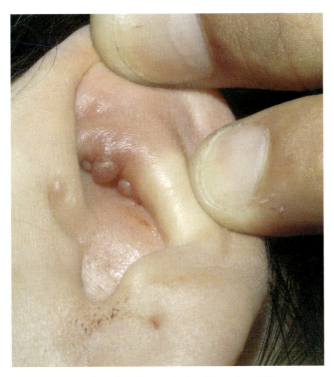

Fig. 15.60. Angiolymphoid hyperplasia with eosinophilia

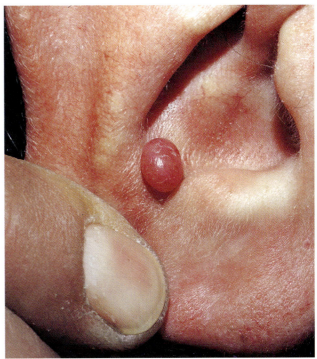

Fig. 15.62. Pyogenic granuloma

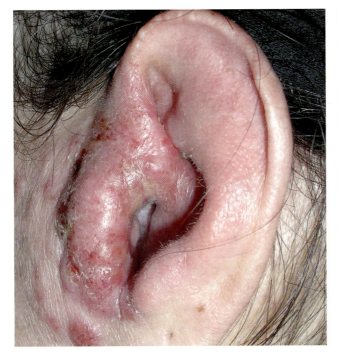

Fig. 15.61. Angiolymphoid hyperplasia with eosinophilia

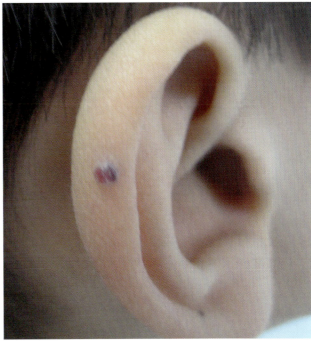

Fig. 15.63. Blue rubber bleb nevus syndrome

highly variable and their surface may be smooth or ulcerated. Lesions may also be located on the trunk, genitalia and oral mucosa. Systemic involvement may be seen especially in the gastrointestinal tract. Highly active antiretroviral therapy can be considered to control AIDS-associated Kaposi's sarcoma. Bacillary angiomatosis can also involve the ear in AIDS patients and manifests as angiomatous nodules. Lymphangioma circumscriptum may be observed on the ear

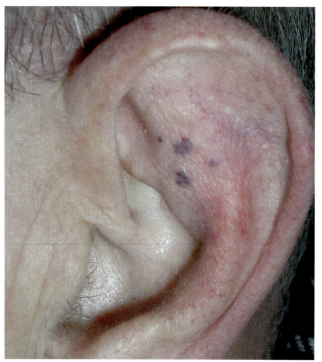

Fig. 15.64. Venous lake

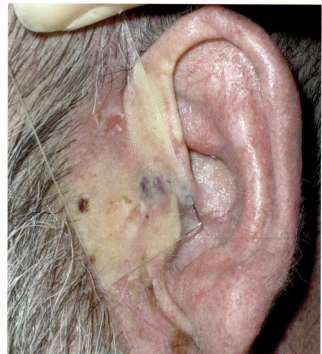

Fig. 15.66. Venous lake

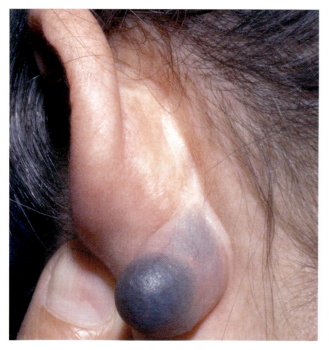

Fig. 15.65. Venous lake

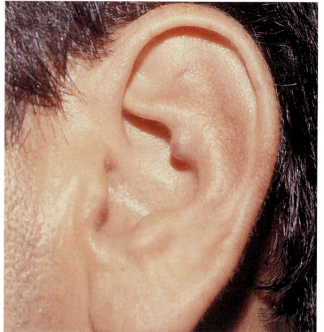

Fig. 15.67. Kaposi's sarcoma

as 2 to 5 mm sized pseudovesicles containing lymph fluid and sometimes occludes the external auditory meatus.

Inflammatory diseases like erythema multiforme, Sweet's syndrome and erythema elevatum diutinum can cause erythematous nodules and plaques on the ears. The most common cause of erythema multiforme is orofacial herpes simplex. The typical target-like lesion is hard to be noticed on pinna (Fig. 15.69). However, there may be accompanying target-like erythematous papules and nodules on the face and extremities. Lesions tend to heal

15 Nodular Lesions

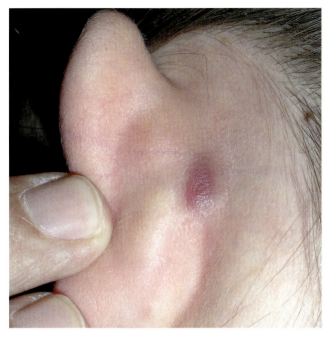

Fig. 15.68. Kaposi's sarcoma

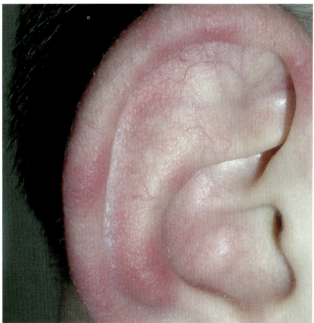

Fig. 15.70. Sweet's syndrome

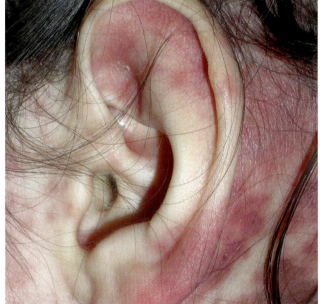

Fig. 15.69. Erythema multiforme

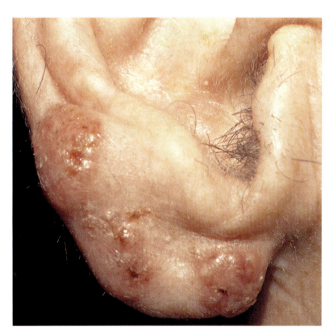

Fig. 15.71. Erythema elevatum diutinum

spontaneously in a few days. Sweet's syndrome presents with sudden-onset erythematous macules, nodules and/or plaques that are warm and tender which may also be seen on the ear as well as anywhere else of the body (Fig. 15.70). Patients tend to be severely ill with high fever. Neutrophilia, leucocytosis and elevated sedimentation rate are the accompanying laboratory findings. When compared to women, the risk of an associated malignancy is higher in men. Lesions heal spontaneously or with systemic therapy such as corticosteroids. However, recurrences may be seen. Erythema elevatum diutinum is a chronic vasculitis involving the extensor surfaces of the extremities and face as well as the ears (Fig. 15.71). This condition can occur in association with hematological malignancies. Soft and mobile reddish brown or violaceous nodules and plaques evolve into firm and fibrotic nodules over time.

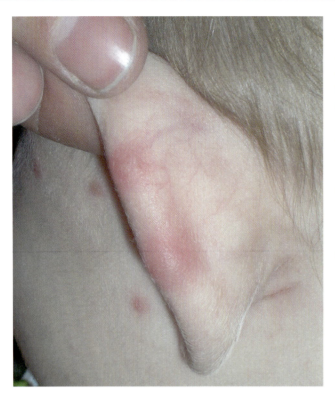

Fig. 15.72. Nodular scabies

The typical sites of granuloma faciale are the nose and the other parts of the face, however ear lesions may occasionally occur, especially on the earlobe. The diagnosis of this chronic inflammatory cutaneous disorder can be confirmed by histopathological examination of the nodules. Rosacea involves the midface most commonly, but sometimes can also be located on the ears. Phymatous rosacea occurs on sites where papulopustular lesions of long duration are seen. Although not as common as on the nose, irregular nodules and plaques with pilosebaceous poral orifices on the surface may be observed on the earlobe (otophyma).

Nodular scabies may be seen as red nodules on the ear as well as on other parts of the body. It may appear during active scabies and persist after other lesions of scabies have healed (Fig 15.72).

16 ■ Granulomatous Lesions

Many spesific chronic infections which cause granulomatous lesions, non-infectious systemic granulomatous diseases, idiopathic cutaneous granulomas and some diseases in which granulomas occur as a reaction to the exogenous factors may involve the ears. The granulomatous lesions of lupus vulgaris have a predilection for earlobes, but can be observed on any part of the ear (Figs. 16.1, 16.2). They can be strictly limited to the ear in some cases. *M. tuberculosis* is thought to reach the ear by haematogenous spread. Reddish brown, soft nodules and plaques tend to be asymptomatic and grow slowly. Neglected or misdiagnosed lesions may enlarge forming huge tumors and cover most of the ear surface (Figs. 16.3, 16.4). Deep infiltration may cause destruction of the ear cartilage (lupus vulgaris mutilans). Treatment with multidrug regimens for tuberculosis is effective against the chronic lesions. However, the earlobe lesions may heal with atrophy and result in disfigurement. Swimming pool granuloma is an atypical mycobacterial infection starting at the site of injury due to the inoculation of *Mycobacterium marinum*. Purple red papulonodular lesions may sometimes be located on the nose and ears as these sites are subjected to physical trauma.

The skin and nervous system are primarily involved in leprosy which is a slowly progressive infection. Facial involvement with numerous granulomatous lesions is typical in lepromatous leprosy. Papules, nodules, plaques or diffuse infiltration on the ears may be prominent (Figs. 16.5-16.8). The earlobes and helix are the common sites, but lesions can appear on any part of the ears. Wrinkled appearance of the ears with other parts of the face is typical. Secondary bacterial infection may cause perichondritis. If not treated with appropriate antibiotics, it can result in cartilage necrosis and scarring. The skin of the earlobe contains many bacilli (*M. leprae*), therefore it is a suitable site for smear investigation even if there are no visible lesions. Leprosy should be treated for a long time with combination therapies including dapson. Multidrug therapy of the patients with infiltrative, tense lesions of the earlobe may result in sagging of the earlobe with loose skin. Granulomatous plaques on the ears can also

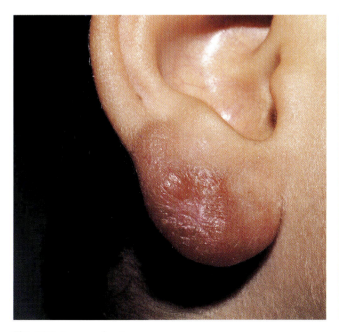

Fig. 16.1. Lupus vulgaris

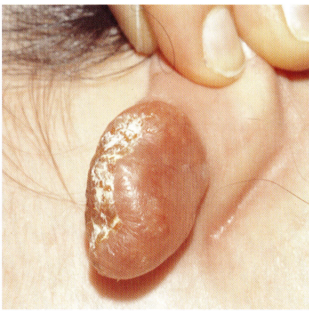

Fig. 16.2. Lupus vulgaris

132 **Ear.** The Importance from a Dermatological Point of View

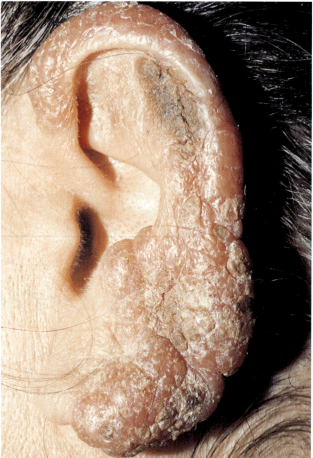

Fig. 16.3. Lupus vulgaris

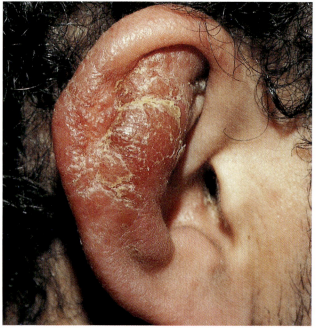

Fig. 16.4. Lupus vulgaris

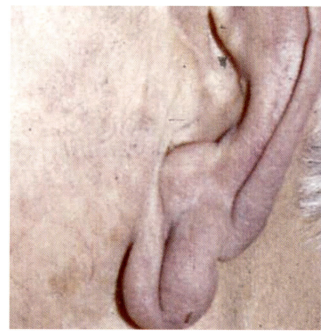

Fig. 16.5. Leprosy

Fig. 16.6. Leprosy

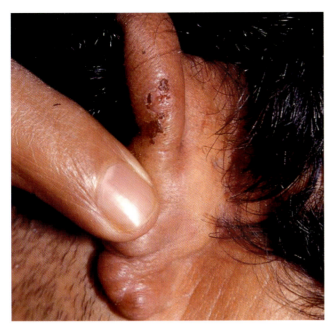

Fig. 16.7. Leprosy

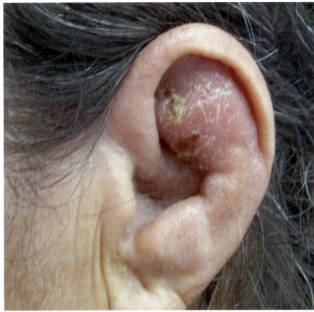

Fig. 16.9. Cutaneous leishmaniasis

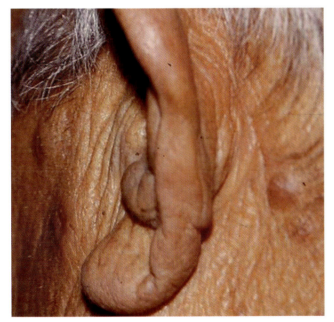

Fig. 16.8. Leprosy

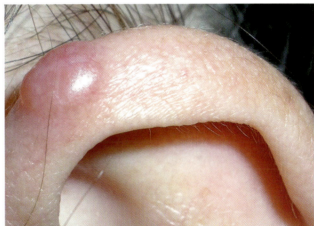

Fig. 16.10. Sarcoidosis

be observed in the late stages or in recurrent lesions of cutaneous leishmaniasis (Fig. 16.9).

Deep mycoses like chromoblastomycosis can cause granulomatous nodules on the ears. Diagnosis depends on the positive tissue culture.

Wegener's granulomatosis more frequently involves the middle and inner ear, but may rarely occur around the ear with nodulo-ulcerative lesions and draining sinuses. Crohn's disease is a chronic granulomatous disease of the bowel causing abscesses and fistula in the perianal area. In metastatic Crohn's disease inflammatory skin lesions in the form of inflammatory plaques may rarely occur on different parts of the body including the ears. The clinical appearance tends to be atypical and histopathological examination shows non-caseating granulomas. Cutaneous lesions of Crohn's disease do not always correlate with intestinal disease activity.

Although rare when compared to nasal involvement, sarcoidosis can also involve the ear (Figs. 16.10, 16.11). Infiltrated plaques are called "lupus pernio", like the nasal lesions. The main sites of involvement on the ear are the earlobe and helix, but lesions of sarcoidosis may occur on any part of the ear. Typical lesions are reddish or purple papules, nodules and plaques with a smooth surface. Enlargement of the earlobes may be prominent in some cases. Patients often have other skin lesions on other parts of the body and also pulmonary involvement. The middle ear and temporal bones

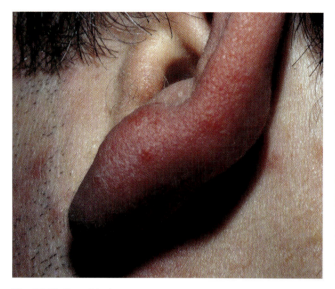

Fig. 16.11. Sarcoidosis

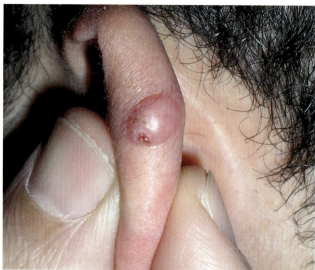

Fig. 16.13. Allergic contact granuloma

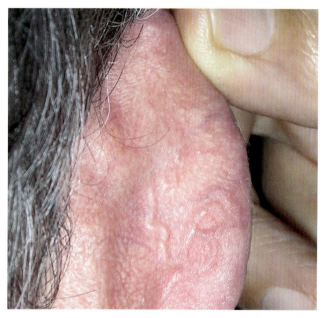

Fig. 16.12. Granuloma annulare

may also rarely be involved. Skin lesions of sarcoidosis respond well to systemic therapy. Although not very often, rheumatoid nodules and granuloma annulare can be observed on the ears. Approximately 20% of patients with rheumatoid arthritis have rheumatoid nodules that mostly appear on the elbows and joints of the hands. However, these granulomatous lesions may sometimes involve the ear, nose and even internal organs such as the lung, pleura, larynx, trachea and meninges. Granuloma annulare may involve only the ear, or auricular lesions sometimes accompany skin lesions on the other sites of the body. Lesions tend to be located mostly on the helix and sometimes at the back side of the ear (Fig. 16.12). Bilateral involvement can sometimes occur. Besides the typical clinical appearance as small grouped papules distributed in annular configuration, granuloma annulare may also present as flesh-coloured nodules on the ears. These lesions do not cause any subjective complaints, they only pose a transient cosmetic problem. Perforating form of granuloma annulare can also develop on the ear.

Acanthoma fissuratum is a granulomatous disease which occurs as a result of constant minor trauma of ill-fitting glasses and usually occurs at the junction of the auricle with the scalp or behind the ear. There is usually a history of wearing new glasses, weeks or a few months prior to the appearance of the lesions. In addition, hearing devices may also be a causative factor. This lesion is characterized by a unilateral 1-2 cm sized pink plaque with a linear groove at the center, but may occasionally be bilateral. It may sometimes be tender. The lesion usually resolves when glasses are changed. Excision may rarely be indicated.

Allergic contact granuloma can occur due to metals applied for ear piercing. It usually develops as papulonodular lesions at sites of piercing on the earlobe and helix (Fig. 16.13). It typically develops 3-4 weeks after this procedure. Positive patch test reaction to the responsible metal confirms the diagnosis.

17 ■ Deformities

The size, shape and exact localization of the ear has minor variations between individuals. Furthermore, the ears may be extremely large (macrotia), small (microtia), sometimes completely absent (anotia) or an extra ear (polyotia) may be present. Some ears may be protruding or sloping forwards. The folds of the ears may also be abnormal like "cup ear" observed in anhidrotic ectodermal dysplasia. The whole spectrum of these abnormalities of the ear is not under the scope of this book. Our aim is to present the abnormalities which are often considered in the differential diagnosis of some dermatological diseases and deformities caused by dermatological diseases or associated with genodermatoses.

All layers of the overlying skin of the ear are relatively thin. Therefore, many diseases of the auricle of either tumoral or inflammatory origin could easily invade the underlying cartilage tissue and cause permanent deformities.

Since the ears are prone to trauma due their protuberant location, traumatic deformities are frequent causes of irregular clefts in the earlobes (torn earlobes). Wearing heavy earrings for a long duration, direct trauma of babies pulling the lobes, and stress from the telephone cords and hairbrushes are major causes of torn earlobes (Fig. 17.1). Sometimes the distal part of the earlobe could be separated into two parts with this traumatic cleft (Fig. 17.2). A torn earlobe poses

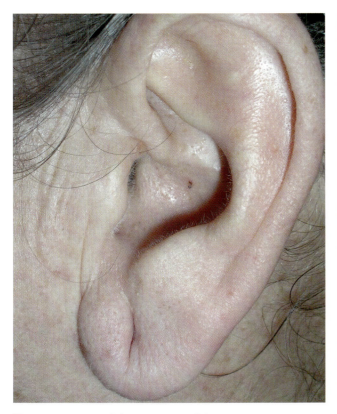

Fig. 17.1. Traumatic deformity. Torn earlobe

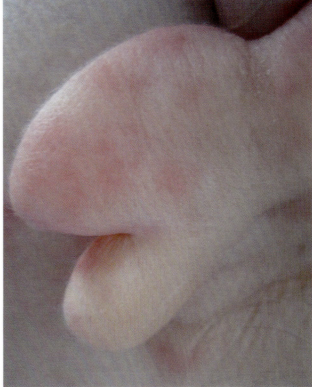

Fig. 17.2. Traumatic deformity. Torn earlobe

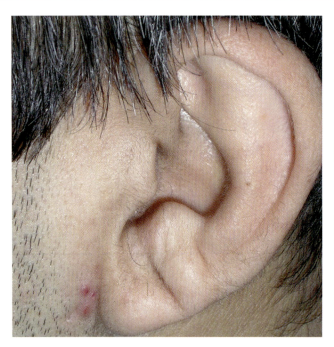

Fig. 17.3. Diagonal earlobe creases

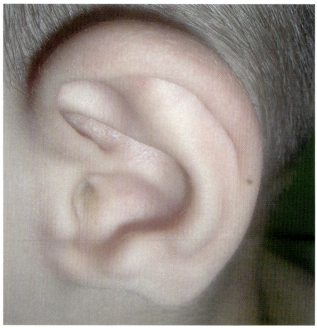

Fig. 17.4. Absent earlobe

a cosmetic problem and can be repaired surgically. Diagonal earlobe creases are bilateral congenital creases which are thought to be associated with coronary artery disease (Fig. 17.3). In Beckwith-Wiedemann syndrome ear creases and posterior helical ear pits can be observed. Typical findings of this disease include nevus flammeus and infantile capillary hemangioma which are localized in the midface, sometimes involving glabella and upper eyelids extending to the nose and upper lips. Other important signs of this disease are macroglossy, organomegaly, omphalocel and somatic gigantism. There is also an increased risk of embriyonic tumors in these patients.

Many genetic diseases with multisystem involvement cause congenital ear deformities. The different location of the ear or its abnormal shape may sometimes give clue to diagnosis. Mental retardation may accompany some of these genodermatoses. Ear anomalies, such as low-set ears and small ears with dysplastic or absent earlobes, may be observed in Down's syndrome (Fig. 17.4). Syringoma, alopecia areata and elastosis perforans serpiginosa are other common dermatological features of this relatively frequent congenital mental retardation syndrome. Branchio-oculo-facial syndrome is a branchial cleft disorder characterized by bilateral cervical, supraauricular defects with overlying aplastic skin (psoriasiform plaques on the lateral sides of the neck along the sternocleidomastoid muscle), early greying of the hair, scalp cysts and auricular pits. Branchial cleft, sinus and cysts may be seen behind the ears. The ears are low-set and posteriorly rotated. There may be malformations of the helix, antihelix and earlobe. Some patients may have accessory tragus. Cleft lip or palate, high arched palate, pseudocleft of the upper lip

are other craniofacial findings. The ocular findings include microophthalmia, anophthalmia, colobomas and nasolacrimal duct stenosis leading to conjunctivitis, otitis and rhinitis.

One of the premature aging syndromes is Hutchinson-Gilford syndrome (progeria) which manifests with craniofacial abnormalities such as frontal bossing, micrognathia, prominent eyes and a beaked nose. The ears are small without earlobes. Patients are mentally normal. Premature atherosclerosis can lead to severe complications. Photosensitivity, subcutaneous fat loss and skin atrophy accompanies Cockayne syndrome with typical thin, beaked nose and large ears ("Mickey Mouse" appearance). The hands and feet of the patients tend to be large. It also causes diffuse demyelination of the central nervous system and peripheral nerves, progressive neurologic deterioration and joint contractures. Ocular findings such as "salt-and-pepper" appearence of retinal pigmention, cataract, sensorineural deafness and mental retardation are other features of this syndrome which causes a short life span. Lymphedema of the extremities, café au lait macules, melanocytic nevi, light-coloured curly hair, ulerythema ophryogenes, and tendency for keloid formation are the typical dermatological features of Noonan syndrome. Other clinical signs include webbed neck, high-arched palate, hypertelorism and micrognathia. The ears are low-set, the helices are thickened and the nasal bridge is depressed. Mental retardation is typical. Cardiovascular findings such as pulmonary valve stenosis, atrial septal defects, and cryptorchidism may also accompany this condition. Hypertelorism and hypotrophy of the malar areas are facial dysmorphic features of Rothmund-Thomson syndrome, but ear deformities are not well-described. There

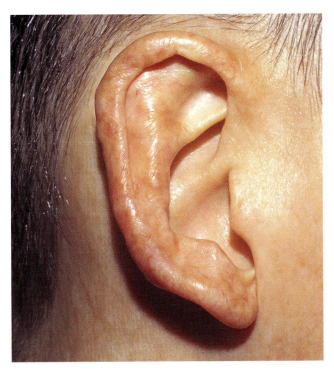

Fig. 17.5. Rothmund-Thomson syndrome

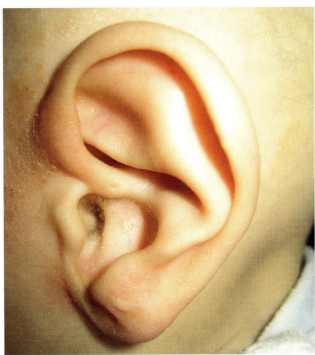

Fig. 17.6. Anhidrotic ectodermal dysplasia

may be skin atrophy on the ears due to photosensitive skin eruption (Fig. 17.5).

Joint hypermobility, hyperextensible skin with "snap-back" elasticity and atrophic scars are the main findings of Ehlers-Danlos syndrome. In the vascular type of this syndrome (Type IV) earlobes are absent. The facial skin is thin and the nose is small. Complications like arterial and gastrointestinal ruptures are potential causes of death in this syndrome. As well as nasal deformity, abnormal ears are also seen in anhidrotic (hypohidrotic) ectodermal dysplasia. Ears are low-set, concha and earlobe may be hypoplastic (Fig. 17.6). Other ear findings include hypoplasia of the ear mucus glands leading to impact cerumen and chronic otitis media. There may be other ear deformities such as cup ear, atypical helical folds, and tragus abnormalities in different types of ectodermal dysplasia. Craniofacial dysmorphism is a typical feature of cardiofacio-cutaneous syndrome in addition to heart defects and ectodermal dysplasia (hair, skin, nail and teeth abnormalities). Low-set ears with helix hyperkeratosis and back-inverted appearance may accompany the nasal deformity. Early identification of cardiac defects and surgical interventions in appropriate cases reduce the morbidity and mortality of this disease.

The size of the ear may be small at birth, and sometimes this is due to an acquired defect caused by tissue loss related to various diseases. Underdevelopment of the external ear associated with complete or partial obstruction of the external auditory canal is named microtia (small ear) (Fig. 17.7). Sometimes a remnant earlobe, tragus or other ear tissue

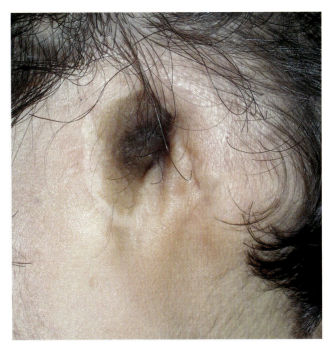

Fig. 17.7. Microtia

is observed. Some patients have facial nerve weakness on the affected size. This abnormality poses a severe cosmetic problem and may accompany other facial abnormalities associated with some syndromes. Implants are used in the treatment (Fig. 17.8). Oculo-auriculo-vertebral spectrum (Goldenhar syndrome) is characterized by epibulber dermoids, hemifacial

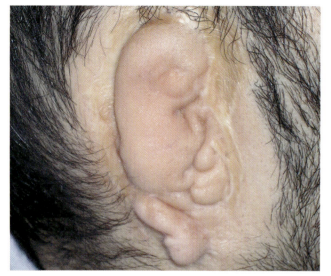

Fig. 17.8. Microtia (after reconstructive surgery)

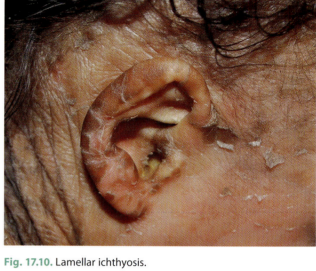

Fig. 17.10. Lamellar ichthyosis.

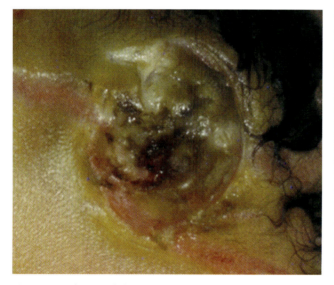

Fig. 17.9. Harlequin ichthyosis. Rudimentary ears

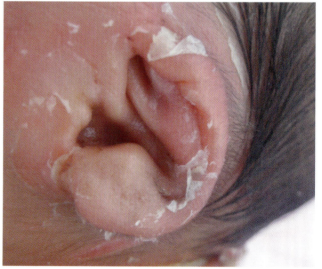

Fig. 17.11. Lamellar ichthyosis.

microsomia, unilateral or bilateral microtia, preauricular tag (accessory tragus), deafness and vertebral abnormalities. The auricular deformities are the diagnostic signs of this syndrome with concomitant brain, gastrointestinal and urogenital system abnormalities. A multidiciplinary approach is advised to avoid complications and manage the systemic complications. In Treacher-Collins syndrome hypoplasia of facial bones, especially in the malar and mandibular bones is seen together with cleft palate, eye abnormalities like coloboma of the lower eyelid and ear abnormalities like microtia, preauricular sinus and accessory tragus. Finlay-Marks syndrome is characterized by nodules on the scalp and underdevelopment of the nipple in addition to ear abnormalities like hypoplastic tragus, antitragus and flattening of the earlobes and antihelix.

Ichthyoses are a heterogenous group of keratinization disorder characterized by a generalized scaling of the skin. The entire body is covered by thick, compact, greyish plates resembling an armour in newborns with harlequin ichthyosis. Typical ear malformations of the patients are absent or rudimentary ears (Fig. 17.9). Gross ectropion, eclabion and "O" shaped mouth are other characteristic facial features. Superinfections and sepsis are life threatening in this type of ichthyosis with high mortality rate. Lamellar ichthyosis is another type of severe ichthyoses, deriving mostly from a collodion-baby presentation (parchment-like membrane covering the entire body surface). The body is covered with large, polygonal, greyish brown and tightly adhered scales. Besides ectropion and eclabion, newborns have everted and deformed ears (Figs. 17.10, 17.11). Ears may sometimes be adhered to the scalp.

Ear deformities can develop after excisions performed for the treatment of basal cell carcinoma and squamous cell

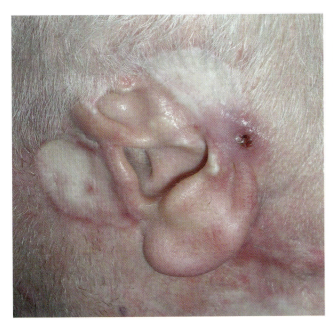

Fig. 17.12. Squamous cell carcinoma. Ear deformity due to surgery

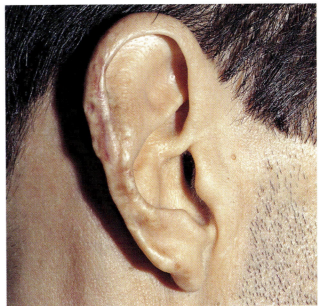

Fig. 17.14. Petrified ear

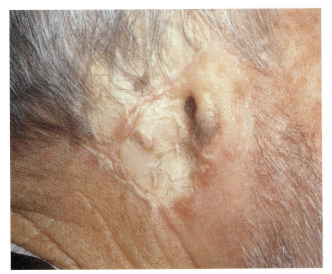

Fig. 17.13. Squamous cell carcinoma. Ear amputation

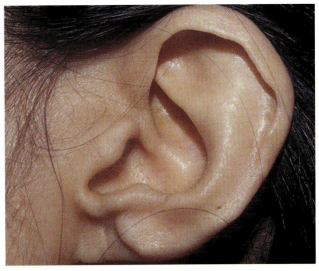

Fig. 17.15. Linear morphea

carcinoma or due to involvement of deep tissues in neglected cases. The ears may become smaller (Fig. 17.12), or anotia (Fig. 17.13) may occur as a result of amputation.

"Petrified ear" is calcification of the auricular cartilage (Fig. 17.14). The auricular cartilage becomes stony-hard and inflexible. It spares the earlobes. There may be no visible changes on the ear. The calcification may be metabolic in cases with elevated calcium and phosporus or dystrophic due to damage or inflammation of the cartilage. The calcification may be caused by various systemic disorders including endocrinopathies or exogenous factors like frostbite, trauma, actinic damage and radiotherapy. In addition, ectopic ossification may also cause a similar clinical picture. Calcification and ossification both could be diagnosed with radiological investigations.

Morphea is the localized form of scleroderma involving both superficial and the deeper layers of the dermis. Linear morphea has a predilection for the forehead and chin but it can also appear on other parts of the head. Mostly being unilateral, the disease can cause loss of subcutaneous tissue in the late stage. When linear morphea involves the ear, the auricle may become smaller due to tissue loss (Fig. 17.15). Another disease causing small auricula is lupus panniculitis. It starts with rubbery-firm, erythematous, nontender nodules and heals with deep depressions due to lipoatrophy. Loss of subcutaneous tissue of the earlobe causes a smaller auricle (Fig. 17.16).

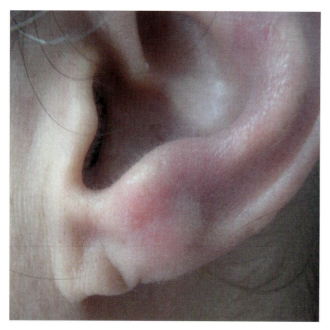

Fig. 17.16. Lupus panniculitis

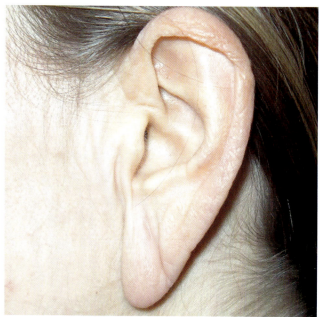

Fig. 17.18. Cutis laxa

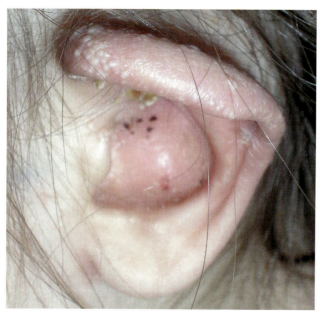

Fig. 17.17. Congenital epidermolysis bullosa

In some photosensitive dermatoses, vesiculobullous lesions which occur after ultraviolet light exposure heal with scarring. Relapsing bullae on the ears cause chronic ulcers, scars and ultimately permanent deformities in congenital erythropoietic porphyria and hepatoerythropoietic porphyria. Erythropoietic protoporphyria starts in childhood with mild photosensitivity and later in life there may be thickening of the facial skin and atrophy on the helix.

Drug use in pregnancy may result in different ear malformations. Thalidomide embryopathia may lead to small, malformed ears, while retinoid embryopathia leads to low-set ears. "Railroad track" ears may be seen in fetal alcohol syndrome. Nasal malformations such as anteverted nares, long philtrum and a flat nasal bridge may also be observed in children who are prenatally exposed to alcohol.

Ear and nose deformities are especially common in "junctional" type of congenital epidermolysis bullosa manifesting with pyloric atresia. In the "dystrophic type" of epidermolysis bullosa, scars due to recurrent bullae may cause adherence between helix and antihelix resulting in permanent deformity (Fig. 17.17). Stenosis of the external auditory canal may also occur.

Earlobes are loose and sagging in congenital or acquired forms of cutis laxa (Fig. 17.18). The acquired form may be generalized or localized to the face and ears. Complications like hernia, diverticles and aortic rupture are life threatening. Earlobes may become loose and sagging after the treatment of infiltrative earlobe lesions of lupus vulgaris and leprosy.

Relapsing polychondritis may cause a "cauliflower-like" appearance of the auricle due to the intensive damage of the cartilage as a result of inflammatory attacks (Fig. 17.19). Infectious chondritis may also cause ear deformity in severe cases due to cartilage necrosis. Wrestler's ear is an acute auricular hematoma (blood collection between the auricular perichondrium and cartilage) developing as a result of traumatic damage to the ear especially among athletes. An initial painless cystic lesion is observed, especially on the anterior part of the auricle. Drainage of the hematoma is required. However, if not freshly drained, the lesion persists and evolves into a firm nodule. Later, formation of fibrous cartilage results in the typical "cauliflower-like" appearance with

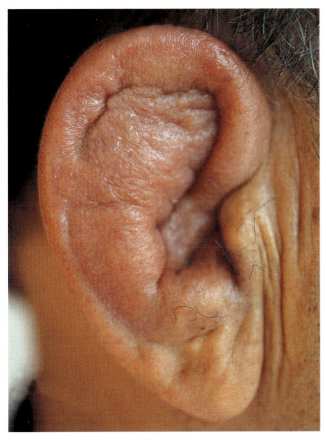

Fig. 17.19. Relapsing polychondritis

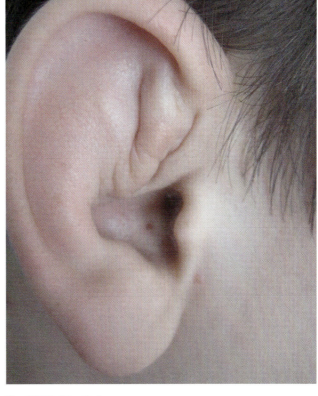

Fig. 17.20. Wrestler's ear

irregular bumpy nodules (Fig. 17.20). Lobomycosis, a deep mycosis, may also cause cauliflower ear in the late stage.

Macrotia (big ear) may be idiopathic or may be a sign of Turner syndrome, Zimmermann-Laband syndrome, Kabuki syndrome and congenital generalized lipoatrophy. Zimmermann-Laband syndrome is characterized by gingival hyperplasia or gingival fibromatosis. Cartilaginous parts of the nose and ears may sometimes be large and soft in these patients. Dysmorphic facial features are characteristic in Kabuki syndrome with multiorgan involvement and common mental retardation. Ears may be large and nasal tip may be depressed. Preauricular pits may accompany. Congenital generalized lipoatrophy (Berardinelli-Seip syndrome) is characterized by loss of buccal fat, coarse facies with gaunt cheeks, large ears, hirsutism and severe acanthosis nigricans. Marked insulin resistant diabetes mellitus, hepatomegaly and genital hypertrophy are among the systemic findings. Mental retardation may accompany.

Benign skin tumors such as nevus flammeus (Fig. 10.18), lymphangioma, congenital giant hairy nevus and neurofibroma may cause asymmetrical enlargement of the ear.

18 ■ Ulcerative Lesions

External physical factors, malignant tumors, infections and vascular diseases are major causes of ear ulcers. Early diagnosis and treatment of these ulcers are very important because secondary infections and invasion to underlying deep tissue may cause serious complications.

Preauricular sinus is not a real ulceration by definition, but presents as a pit located typically on the preauricular area. Frostbite begins on acral sites including the ears. Vesicles and bullae may evolve into ischemic necrosis and various degrees of tissue destruction may occur due to this cold dermatosis. Herpes simplex infection may cause ulcers on the ears, especially in immunocompromised patients.

Basal cell carcinoma (Figs. 18.1-18.3) and squamous cell carcinoma (Figs. 12.22, 18.4, 18.5) are the main underlying causes of chronic ulcers on this area. The ulceration of basal cell carcinoma is usually hidden by a crust at the center of the nodule with slightly raised and rolled margins. On the other hand, the ulceration of squamous cell carcinoma grows more rapidly than that of basal cell carcinoma and may cover the entire surface of the tumor. The metastatic potential of squamous cell carcinoma on the ear is relatively

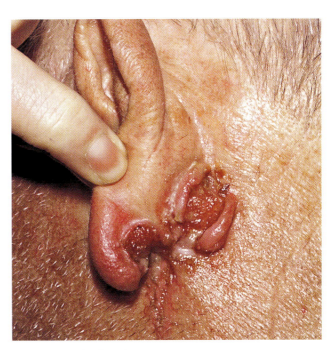

Fig. 18.2. Basal cell carcinoma

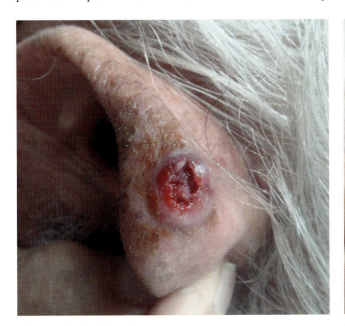

Fig. 18.1. Basal cell carcinoma

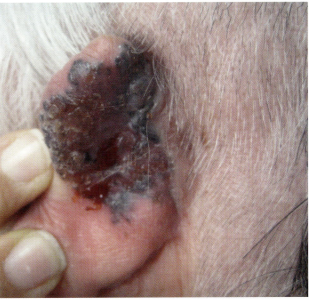

Fig. 18.3. Basal cell carcinoma

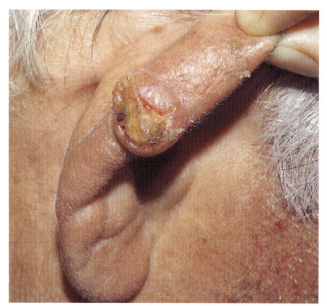

Fig. 18.4. Squamous cell carcinoma

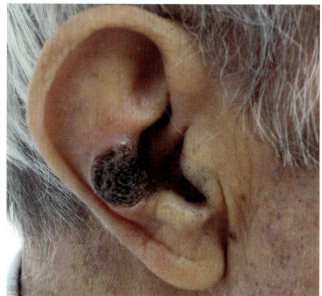

Fig. 18.6. Lymphomatoid papulosis

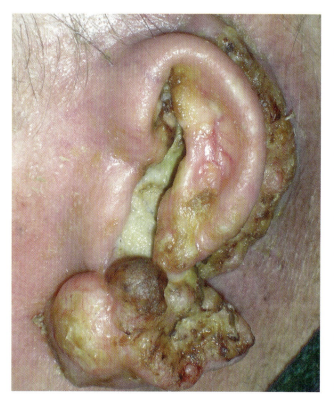

Fig. 18.5. Squamous cell carcinoma

high. Radiotherapy for the ear tumors may result with scarring and radionecrosis. Atypical fibroxanthoma, malignant melanoma, Kaposi's sarcoma and angiosarcoma may also cause ear ulceration in the late stages. Nodulo-ulcerative lesions of lymphomatoid papulosis with sudden onset may be observed on the ears (Fig. 18.6). A history of reccurrent but spontaneously-healing lesions in different parts of the body including ears is typical for this type of CD30+ lymphopropherative disease.

Cutaneous leishmaniasis may be located on the ears although not as frequent as the face. A painless solitary ulcerated nodule with adherent crust is the typical clinical appearance of this parasitical dermatosis which is encountered endemically in several regions of the world (Figs. 18.7, 18.8). Chiclero ulcer is a subtype of the New World leishmaniasis seen mostly in the Central and South American countries, especially in farmers harvesting chicle from the sapodilla tree for chewing gum production in highly humid forests. It causes a deep painful ulceration on the ear, mostly on the helix which may result in deformity due to the destruction of the ear cartilage.

Pyoderma gangrenosum should be considered in the differential diagnosis of persistent ulcers with variable size on the ear and preauricular area. A histopathological examination can be helpful for diagnosis. Purpura fulminans, which is a typical finding of disseminated intravascular coagulation, can be observed on acral regions such as the ears and nose in addition to extremities. Lesions start suddenly in the form of purpura, may enlarge rapidly and result in sharply demarcated deep ulcerations with adherent necrotic crusts. The general health of patients is poor, and there is a high risk of mortality.

18 Ulcerative Lesions 145

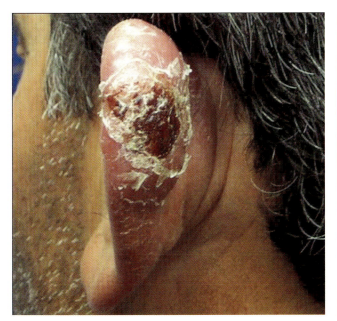

Fig. 18.7. Cutaneous leishmaniasis

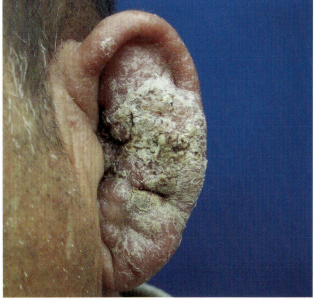

Fig. 18.8. Cutaneous leishmaniasis

19 ■ Hypertrichosis

Localized changes of hair are also important in the diagnosis of some dermatological diseases like in the case of elementary lesions. The ear consists of hair follicles in different parts, and overgrowth of hair may be present in some congenital and acquired entities. Ear hypertrichosis may be a feature of diseases causing diffuse hypertrichosis, or may be an isolated finding. In the latter case, there may be an association with underlying tumoral lesions, or the presentation solely bases on overgrowth of hair. Increased hairs may be of lanugo type (fine, soft, unmedullated, light-coloured) or terminal type (thick, medullated, pigmented). Hairy pinna is a variation of human hair with age (Figs. 19.1, 19.2). It usually becomes evident in the third or fourth decade and almost exclusively affects men. There is a possible hereditary tendency. Coarse terminal hairs typically grow on tragus bilaterally. Some patients have hypertrichosis, especially on the lower part of the helix and some in both localizations. This type of hypertrichosis does not generally have any underlying cause but it poses a cosmetic problem. On the other hand, some AIDS patients may show acquired hairy pinna in addition to eyelash trichomegaly.

Excessive hair growth causing severe cosmetic problems together with dysmorphic facial features are present in Ambras syndrome. Hypertrichosis appears at birth on the whole body and is more prominent on the shoulders, face, nose and ears. It spares only the palmoplantar and genital regions. External auditory meatus would not be seen due to long and thick terminal hairs. Congenital hypertrichosis lanuginosa manifests with an increase in lanugo type of hair on nearly all parts of the body. Ear deformities, dental abnormalities and gingival fibromatosis are other manifestations. Acquired hypertrichosis lanuginosa is an ominous sign of internal malignancies. It

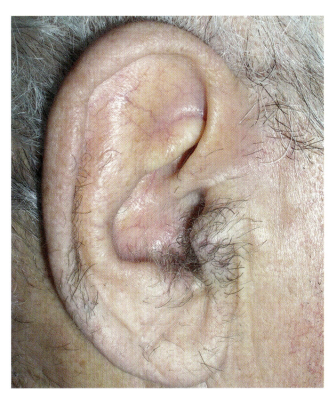

Fig. 19.1. Hairy pinna

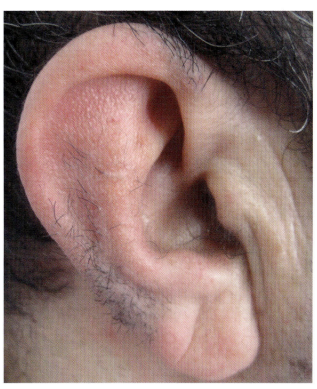

Fig. 19.2. Hairy pinna

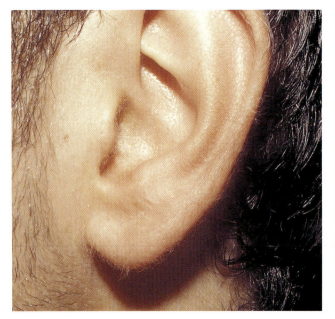

Fig. 19.3. Acquired hypertrichosis lanuginosa

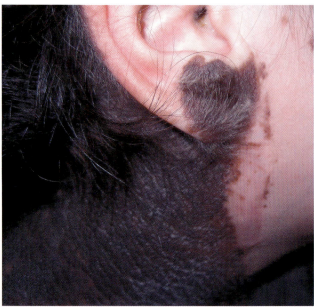

Fig. 19.5. Congenital giant hairy nevus

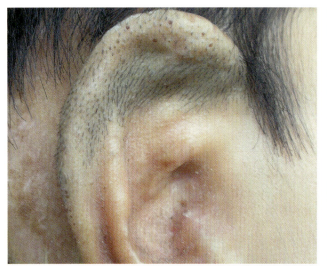

Fig. 19.4. Hypertrichosis after reconstructive ear surgery

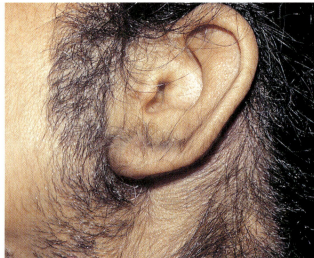

Fig. 19.6. Plexiform neurofibroma

is seen mostly in adulthood as a sudden hair increase on the face together with the ears (Fig. 19.3). After the treatment of underlying malignancy, the hair content of the patients decreases. Hypertrichosis of the ears can also be seen in children of diabetic mothers. The hair growth is mild at birth, but becomes evident over time.

During the course of porphyria cutanea tarda bilateral hypertrichosis of the ears may occur. Hypertrichosis of the face, recurrent bullae and atrophic scars are other features of this metabolic disease. Hypertrichosis related to systemic drugs such as cyclosporine, phenytoin and minoxidil may also be prominent on the ears in addition to the face. Topically applied minoxidil may cause hair growth on the ears, too. Hypertrichosis also involving the external auditory canal regresses after discontinuation of the responsible drug. The excessive hair on the external auditory canal associated with either hairy pinna or drug-related hypertrichosis may form a bulk with mixture of cerumen affecting the ventilation and create vulnerability to external otitis. Hair growth may also occur after reconstructive surgery for auricular malformations like microtia and poses a cosmetic problem (Fig. 19.4).

Ear hypertrichosis due to the underlying tumoral lesions is typically unilateral. There can be excessive hair on congenital giant hairy nevi involving the ears (Fig. 19.5). The lesion is present at birth, and terminal hairs increase as the patient ages. The underlying nevus is mostly a darkly pigmented, slightly elevated, large plaque with a pebbled surface. Hairs are coarse and dark. Hypertrophy of the earlobe is common in these patients. Plexiform neurofibroma may also be located on the ear with typically overlying pigmentation and increased terminal hairs (Fig. 19.6). The large mass of this acquired tumor may be soft and pendulous. The ear may be enlarged and malpositioned. It is an important diagnostic criterion for neurofibromatosis type I and carries a risk of malignant transformation.

Reference Books

1. Bolognia JL, Jorizzo JL, Rapini RP (2003) Dermatology. Mosby, Spain
2. Bornhill RL, Fitzpatrick TB, Fondrey K et al (1995) Color Atlas and Synopsis of Pigmented Lesions. Mc Graw-Hill, USA
3. Braun-Falco O, Plewig G, Wolff HH, Burgdorf WHC (2000) Dermatology, 2nd edn. Springer, Berlin, Germany
4. Burns T, Breathnach NC, Griffiths C (2004) Rook's Textbook of Dermatology, 7th edn. Blackwell, Italy
5. Caputo R (1998) Text Atlas of Histiocytic Syndromes, A Dermatological Perspective. Martin Dunitz, UK
6. Caputo R, Tadini G (2006) Atlas of Genodermatoses. Taylor & Francis, Spain
7. Cerroni L, Gatter K, Kerl H (2004) An Illustrated Guide to Skin Lymphoma, 2nd edn. Blackwell, India
8. du Vivier A (2002) Atlas of Clinical Dermatology, 3rd edn. Elsevier, Spain
9. Elewski BE, Hughey LC, Parsons ME (2005) Differential Diagnosis in Dermatology. Elsevier Mosby, China
10. Eliot H, Ghatan Y (2002) Dermatological Differential Diagnosis and Pearls, 2nd edn. The Parthenon Publishing Group, USA
11. Gleeson M, Burton M, Clarke R et al (2008) Scott-Brown's Otorhinolaryngology, Head and Neck Surgery, 7th edn. Hodder Arnold, UK
12. Hawke M, Bingham B, Stammberger H, Benjamin B (2002) Diagnostic Handbook of Otorhinolaryngology, 2nd edn. Martin Dunitz, UK
13. James WD, Berger TG, Elston DM (2006) Andrews' Diseases of the Skin. Clinical Dermatology, 10th edn. Elsevier, Canada
14. Mac Kie RM (1989) Skin Cancer. Martin Dunitz, London, UK
15. Mallory SB (2006) An Illustrated Dictionary of Dermatologic Syndromes, 2nd edn. Taylor and Francis, St. Louis, USA
16. Marks R (2007) Facial Skin Disorders. Informa Healthcare, India
17. Paller AS, Mancini AJ (2006) Hurwitz Clinical Pediatric Dermatology, A Textbook of Skin Disorders of Childhood and Adolescence, 3rd edn. Elsevier Saunders, China
18. Rigel DS, Friedman RJ, Dzubow LM et al (2005) Cancer of the Skin. Elsevier, China
19. Schneiderman PI, Grossman ME (2006) A Clinician's Guide to Dermatologic Differential Diagnosis. Informa Healthcare, UK
20. Spitz JL (2006) Genodermatoses. A Clinical Guide to Genetic Skin Disorders, 2nd edn. Lippincott Williams & Wilkins, USA
21. Weinberg S, Prose NS, Kristal L (2008) Color Atlas of Pediatric Dermatology, 4th edn. McGraw Hill Medical, China
22. White GM, Cox NH (2006) Diseases of the Skin, A Color Atlas and Text, 2nd edn. Elsevier-Mosby, Philadelphia, USA

Index

A
Abscess, 13, 34, 89, 133
Absent earlobe, 136
Acantholytic dyskeratosis, 42
Acanthoma fissuratum, 57, 134
Acanthosis nigricans, 4, 64–65, 141
Accessory tragus, 117, 136, 138
Acne vulgaris, 13, 35, 64, 103, 114
Acquired hypertrichosis lanuginosa, 147–148
Acrochordon, 28, 29, 65
Acrodermatitis enteropathica, 19, 94
Acrodynia, 7
Acrogeria, 67
Acrokeratosis paraneoplastica, 23, 102
Acromegaly, 105
Actinic keratosis, 4, 17, 24, 61, 100–102, 121
Actinic prurigo, 15, 89
Actinic reticuloid, 109
Actinomycosis, 42
Acute auricular hematoma, 140
Acute graft versus host disease, 79
Acute hemorrhagic edema, 81
Acute myeloid leukemia, 78
Addison's disease, 77, 105
Adenocarcinoma, 97, 118
Adenoid cystic carcinoma, 118
Adult colloid milium, 33
Adult progeria, 67
AIDS, 19, 34, 47, 69, 127, 147
Albright syndrome, 105
Alkaptonuria, 3
Allergic contact granuloma, 134
Allergic eczematous contact dermatitis, 17, 92
Allergic rhinitis, 35, 67
Allergic salute, 67
Alopecia areata, 136
Alopecia mucinosa, 93
Alopecia, 19, 23, 63, 64, 73, 93, 99
Ambras syndrome, 64, 147
Amelanotic malignant melanoma, 70, 113
Amiadarone, 3
Amyloidosis, 48, 105
Aneurysm, 80
Angioedema, 80
Angiofibroma, 29, 108
Angiolipoleiomyoma, 116
Angiolymphoid hyperplasia with eosinophilia, 124
Angiomatous macule, 7, 8, 77, 82
Angiomyolipoma, 30, 115
Angiosarcoma, 8, 49, 71, 144
Anhidrotic ectodermal dysplasia, 31, 63, 135, 137
Anophthalmia, 136
Anosmia, 41
Anotia, 135, 139
Anthrax, 86
Antimalarial drug, 3, 77
Aort coarctation, 45
Aort rupture, 140
Apert syndrome, 64
Aplasia cutis congenita, 64
Apocrine hidrocystoma, 116
Ara-C ears, 78
Argyria, 4, 77
Arteriovenous malformation, 47, 124
Arthritis, 105
Arthropathy, 4, 119
Aspergillosis, 42, 87
Asphyxia, 80
Ataxia telangiectasia, 82
Atherosclerosis, 67, 136
Atopic dermatitis, 86, 93, 97
Atopic salute, 67
Atrial septal defect, 136
Atrophoderma vermiculatum, 63
Atypical fibroxanthoma, 121, 144
Atypical mycobacterial infection, 131
Auricular pseudocyst, 114

B
B cell chronic lymphocytic leukemia, 119
Bacillary angiomatosis, 46, 127
Bacillus anthracis, 86
Bartonella henselae, 13
Basal cell adenoma, 116
Basal cell carcinoma, 27, 31–32, 39, 41, 44, 49, 57,
    60, 64–65, 67, 69, 70, 114, 116, 120, 123, 138, 143
Basaloid follicular hamartoma syndrome, 31–32
Bazex syndrome, 23, 102
Bazex-Dupré-Christol syndrome, 32, 64
Beaked nose, 21, 67, 136
Beak-like nose, 64, 66–67
Beckwith-Wiedemann syndrome, 136
Behçet's disease, 80
Benign cephalic histiocytosis, 119
Berardinelli-Seip syndrome, 141
Big ear, 141
Bird-like face, 67
Birt-Hogg-Dubé syndrome, 28, 107
Bitemporal constriction, 65
Blackhead, 35
Blastomycosis, 42, 118

151

Bloodhound-like face, 64
Bloom's syndrome, 7, 64, 80
Blue nevus, 38, 112
Blue rubber bleb nevus syndrome, 125
Bonnet-Dechaume-Blanc syndrome, 47
Borrelia burgdorferi, 119
Bowen's disease, 39, 121
Brachycephaly, 64
Branchio-oculo-facial syndrome, 136
Branchio-oto-renal syndrome, 115
Breast cancer, 42
Bronchiectasia, 60
Brooke-Spiegler syndrome, 28, 107, 116, 117
Bulbous nose, 66
Bullous pemphigoid, 14, 88
Burn, 4, 78, 80

C
Café au lait macule, 136
Calcified epithelioma, 51
Calcifying epithelioma of Malherbe, 43
Calcinosis cutis, 105
Carcinoma of the parotid gland, 121
Cardiac abnormalities, 64, 100
Cardiac rhabdomyoma, 30
Cardiofacio-cutaneous (CFC) syndrome, 65, 100, 137
Carney complex, 112
Carpal tunnel syndrome, 48
Caseation necrosis, 54
Cataract, 63, 67, 136
Cat scratch disease, 13
Cauliflower ear, 118–119, 140–141
Cavernous sinus thrombosis, 13
CD30+ lymphoproliferative disorders, 72, 144
Cellulitis, 7, 34, 80, 102
Cerebellar ataxia, 82
Cerebral artery abnormality, 45
Ceruminoma, 118
Chancre, 69
Cherry angioma, 33
Chicken pox, 11
Chiclero ulcer, 144
Chilblain lupus, 79
Chilblains, 108
Chloracne, 103
Chondritis, 63, 80–81, 140
Chondrodermatitis nodularis helicis, 103–104
Chondrodysplasia punctata, 63
Chondroid syringoma, 43, 116
Chordoma, 42
Chromoblastomycosis, 133
Chronic bullous dermatosis of childhood, 14
Chronic graft versus host disease, 66
Chronic liver failure, 33
Chronic lupoid leishmaniasis, 53
Chronic mucocutaneous candidiasis, 42
Chronic myeloid leukemia, 119
Chronic otitis, 120, 137
Chronic radiodermatitis, 24
Cicatricial alopecia, 63–64
Cicatricial pemphigoid, 61, 88
Cleft lip, 65, 136
Cleft palate, 65, 138
Clofazimine, 3, 54
Cocaine abuse, 24, 62, 73
Cockayne syndrome, 67, 136

Coffin-Siris syndrome, 65
Cold dermatosis, 82, 143
Collagen nevus, 29
Collarate-like scales, 95
Collodion-baby, 138
Coloboma, 136, 138
Colon polyp, 30
Comedone, 13, 15, 35, 49, 67, 103, 114
Compound nevus, 112
Congenital calcinosis cutis, 105
Congenital erythropoietic porphyria, 15, 61, 140
Congenital generalized lipoatrophy, 141
Congenital giant hairy nevus, 111, 141, 148
Congenital hypertrichosis lanuginosa, 147
Congenital melanocytic nevus, 37, 111
Congenital syphilis, 62
Conjunctivitis, 33, 136
Conradi-Hünermann-Happle syndrome, 63
Contact dermatitis, 17, 18, 92
Cornu cutaneum, 24
Coronary artery disease, 136
Costello syndrome, 51
Cotrimoxazole, 3
Cowden syndrome, 30, 107
Craniosynostosis, 64
CREST syndrome, 9, 33, 66, 105
Cri du chat syndrome, 118
Crohn's disease, 133
Crusted scabies, 100
Cryofibrinogenemia, 108
Cryoglobulinemia, 82
Cryotherapy, 118
Cryptococcosis, 34, 49, 103
Cryptorchidism, 118, 136
Cup ear, 135, 137
Cutaneous horn, 24, 101
Cutaneous leishmaniasis, 53, 62, 69, 133, 144
Cutaneous leukemia, 41
Cutaneous metastasis, 46
Cutaneous T cell lymphoma, 40
Cutis laxa, 63, 65, 140
Cyclosporine, 30, 35, 110, 148
Cyclosporine-induced folliculodystrophy, 35, 110
Cylindroma, 28, 43, 116
Cyrano nose, 45, 46
Cystadenoma, 116
Cytarabine, 78
Cytosine arabinoside, 78

D
D-penicillamine, 110
Dapson, 131
Darier's disease, 23, 99
Darwin tubercle, 118
Deafness, 23, 62, 66, 136, 138
Deletion 5p syndrome, 118
Demodex folliculorum, 13
Demodicosis, 13
Dermatitis artefacta, 73
Dermatitis herpetiformis, 87
Dermatoheliosis, 49
Dermatomyositis, 79, 105
Dermatophytosis, 92
Dermochondrocorneal dystrophy, 30
Dermoid cyst, 37, 51, 69
Desmoplastic malignant melanoma, 38, 113

Developmental delay, 100
Diabetes insipidus, 33
Diabetes mellitus, 109, 141
Diagonal earlobe crease, 136
Diarrhea, 19
Diascopy, 54
Diltiazem, 77
Discoid lupus erythematosus, 6, 20, 60, 77, 95
Disseminated intravascular coagulation, 144
Diverticle, 140
Dolicocephalia, 64
Donohue syndrome, 64
Down's syndrome, 64, 110, 136
Drug-induced hyperpigmentation, 3
Drug-related hypertrichosis, 148
Dwarfism, 7
Dystopia canthorum, 66
Dystrophic calcification, 105

E
Earlobe rhagade, 93
Early congenital syphilis, 62
Eccrine hidrocystoma, 30, 107
Eccrine spiradenoma, 116
Eclabion, 138
Ectodermal dysplasia, 65
Ectopic ossification, 139
Ectrodactily, 65
Ectropion, 138
Eczema herpeticum, 86
Eczema, 17, 86, 91–93
Eczematization, 19, 94
Eczematous drug reaction, 93
EEC syndrome, 65
Ehlers-Danlos syndrome, 67, 137
Elastosis perforans serpiginosa, 110, 136
Elastotic nodules of the ear, 104
Elephantiasis nostras verrucosa, 102
Elf ear, 118
Elf like facies, 64
Encephalitis, 73
Encephalocele, 37
Eosinophilia, 124
Ephelide, 4
Epibulber dermoid, 137
Epicanthal fold, 118
Epidermal growth factor receptor (EGFR) antagonists induced drug eruption, 13
Epidermal nevus, 102
Epidermal nevus syndrome, 102
Epidermodysplasia verruciformis, 35
Epidermoid cyst, 30–31, 43, 114
Epidermolysis bullosa, 61, 88, 140
Epidermolytic hyperkeratosis, 99
Epistaxis, 14, 41, 47, 53, 71, 97
Epithelioma adenoides cysticum, 28
Erysipelas, 7, 69
Erythema elevatum diutinum, 128–129
Erythema infectiosum, 78
Erythema multiforme, 14, 128
Erythroderma, 97
Erythrodontia, 15
Erythromelalgia, 81
Erythromelanosis follicularis faciei, 79
Erythropoietic protoporphyria, 7, 140
Espundia, 62

Ethyl chloride, 85
External otitis, 86–87, 89, 97, 148
Extramammary Paget's disease, 97

F
Facial dysmorphism, 59, 63, 65
Facial nerve paralysis, 87, 121
Favre-Racouchot syndrome, 48
Fetal alcohol syndrome, 140
Fibroadenoma, 51
Fibrofolliculoma, 28, 107
Fibrous papule of the face, 27–28
Fibrous papule of the nose, 27
Fifth disease, 78
Filiform verruca, 24, 101
Finlay-Marks syndrome, 138
Fixed drug eruption, 3
Flu, 12, 17
5-Fluorouracil 17
Flushing, 78
Focal dermal hypoplasia, 64
Follicular atrophoderma, 32, 64
Follicular mucinosis, 93
Folliculitis, 7, 12, 86
François syndrome, 30
Freckle, 4
Frontal bossing, 60, 63, 136
Frostbite, 80, 85, 105, 139, 143
Furuncle, 13, 86

G
Gangosa, 62
Gastrointestinal carcinoma, 7, 29
Gentamycin, 92
Gigantism, 136
Gingival fibromatosis, 141, 147
Gingival hyperplasia, 141
Glaucoma, 8
Glomerulonephritis, 63, 86
Goitre, 107
Goldenhar syndrome, 117, 137
Goltz syndrome, 64
Gorlin syndrome, 31–32, 60, 65
Gottron syndrome, 67
Gout, 104–105
Granuloma annulare, 134
Granuloma faciale, 47–48, 130
Granulomatous periorificial dermatitis, 57
Granulosis rubra nasi, 11
Graves disease, 107
Greek warrior helmet appearance, 64
Growth retardation, 15, 64–65, 67
Gumma,
Günther's disease, 15, 61

H
Hairy pinna, 147–148
Hand-Schüller-Christian disease, 33
Harlequin ichthyosis, 138
Hearing loss, 66, 85, 89, 115, 118, 121, 124
Hebra nose, 65
Hemangioma, 44–46, 49, 71, 82, 107, 123–125, 136
Hematoma auris, 118
Hematuria, 97
Hemifacial microsomia, 137–138
Hemophagocytic syndrome, 71

Henoch-Schönlein purpura, 81–82
Hepatoerytropoietic porphyria, 140
Hereditary hemorrhagic telangiectasia, 9
Herpes gladiatorum, 86
Herpes simplex infection, 7, 11, 69, 86, 128, 143
Hidradenoma of the external auditory canal, 118
High-arched palate, 136
Hippopotamus nose, 65
Hirsutism, 64–65, 141
Histoplasmosis, 42, 72
HIV infection, 8, 86, 126
Hobnail hemangioma, 46
Hook-like nose, 64
Human papilloma virus (HPV), 24, 34
Huriez syndrome, 9
Hurler syndrome, 63
Hutchinson-Gilford syndrome, 67, 136
Hutchinson sign, 12
Hutchinson's teeth, 62
Hydradenitis suppurativa, 89
Hydroa vacciniforme, 14, 89
Hyperhidrosis, 11
Hyperimmunoglobulinemia-E syndrome, 65, 93
Hyperlipidemic, 105
Hyperpigmentation, 3–4, 6, 77
Hyperpyrexia, 63
Hypertelorism, 60, 65, 136
Hypertension, 7, 81
Hyperthyroidism, 33
Hypertrichosis, 15, 64, 147–148
Hypertrophic scar, 51, 118–119
Hyperuricemia, 105
Hypogonadism, 7
Hypohidrotic ectodermal dysplasia, 63, 137
Hypohydrosis, 32, 64
Hypospadias, 118
Hypotrichosis, 32, 64

I
Ichthyosiform erythroderma, 63
Ichthyosis, 23, 99, 138
Idiopathic thrombocytopenic purpura, 82
Imiquimod, 17
Impetiginization, 86
Impetigo, 12, 86
Impetigo contagiosa, 12
Infantile capillary hemangioma, 44–46, 71, 123–124, 136
Infantile hemorrhagic edema, 81
Infantile spasm, 29
Infantile systemic hyaline fibromatosis, 106
Inflammatory bowel disease, 81
Insect bite, 110
In situ carcinoma, 39, 101
Interstitial keratitis, 62
Intertrigo, 93
Intracranial calcification, 8
Intradermal nevus, 37, 112
Ipsilateral microphtalmy, 45
Iris heterochromia, 66
Irritant contact dermatitis, 17
Isolated mastocytoma, 123

J
Jessner-Kanof disease, 119
Junctional nevus, 111
Juvenile colloid milium, 33, 106

Juvenile dermatomyositis, 105
Juvenile hyaline fibromatosis, 30, 106
Juvenile melanoma, 38
Juvenile spring eruption, 88
Juvenile xanthogranuloma, 44, 46, 119

K
Kabuki syndrome, 141
Kaposi's sarcoma, 8, 46, 126–127, 144
Keloid, 51, 118–119, 136
Keloidal blastomycosis, 118
Keratitis, 12, 23
Keratoacanthoma, 42, 70, 101, 121
Keratosis pilaris, 100
KID syndrome, 23, 99
Kimura disease, 125
Kindler syndrome, 66–67
Klebsiella pneumoniae spp. rhinoscleromatis, 55
Klippel-Trenaunay-Weber syndrome, 46

L
LAMB syndrome, 112
Lamellar ichthyosis, 138
Langerhans cell histiocytosis, 19, 33, 92, 119
Leishmaniasis, 53, 62, 69, 133, 144
Leishmania tropica, 69
Lentigines syndromes, 77
Lentigo maligna, 4
Lentigo malignant melanoma, 4, 38, 113
Lentigo simplex, 77
Lentigo solaris, 4
LEOPARD syndrome, 77
Leprechaunism, 64
Lepromatous leprosy, 62, 131
Leprosy, 3, 53, 62, 69, 131, 140
Lesch-Nyhan syndrome, 105
Lethal midline granuloma, 71
Leukemia, 7, 41, 78
Lichen amyloidosis, 105
Lichen planus, 4, 77
Lichen planus pemphigoides, 88
Lichen planus pigmentosus, 4
Linear ichthyosiform erythroderma, 63
Linear IgA dermatosis, 14, 87
Linear morphea, 139
Lignous conjunctivitis, 33
Lignous periodontitis, 33
Lipoatrophy, 60
Lipodystrophy, 64
Lipoid proteinosis, 105
Lipoma, 107, 115
Lobomycosis, 118, 141
Low-set ear, 136–137, 140
Lung cancer, 42
Lupus miliaris disseminatus faciei, 35, 109–110
Lupus panniculitis, 60, 139
Lupus pernio, 56, 133
Lupus profundus, 60
Lupus vulgaris, 53–54, 59, 131, 140
Lupus vulgaris mutilans, 131
Lyme disease, 119
Lymphangioma, 46, 141
Lymphangioma circumscriptum, 127
Lymphangiomyomatosis, 30
Lymphedema, 102
Lymphocytic infiltration of the skin, 119

Lymphocytoma cutis, 39–40, 118
Lymphomatoid papulosis, 40–41, 72, 144

M
Macrocephaly, 63, 65
Macroglossia, 48, 63, 136
Macrotia, 135, 141
Maculopapular drug eruption, 78
Maffucci syndrome, 46
MAGIC syndrome, 80
Malignant blue nevus, 114
Malignant external otitis, 87
Malignant melanoma, 4, 38, 70, 112–114, 144
Marginal zone lymphoma, 40, 119
Massive lymphadenopathy with sinus histiocytosis, 33
Median nasal dermoid fistule, 37
Medullary thyroid carcinoma, 30
Melanocytic nevus, 37–38, 111–112
Melasma, 3
MEN-2B syndrome, 30
Meningioma, 73
Meningitis, 34
Mental retardation, 29, 63–66, 105, 118, 136, 141
Merkel cell carcinoma, 41, 121
Metageria, 67
Metastatic Crohn's disease, 133
Metastatic malignant melanoma, 113
Mickey Mouse appearance, 136
Microcephaly, 64, 66, 118
Microcystic adnexal carcinoma, 41
Micrognathia, 118, 136
Microophtalmia, 136
Microtia, 135, 137–138, 148
Migraine, 81
Milia, 15, 30–32, 64, 67, 88, 114, 116
Milia an plaque, 114
Minoxidil, 148
Mixed connective tissue disorder, 21
Mixed tumor of skin, 43
Mohs' microsurgery, 120
Molluscum contagiosum, 34, 103
Morbilliform drug eruption, 78
Morphea, 139
Morpheaform type of basal cell carcinoma, 39, 67
Mucormycosis, 72, 87
Muir-Torre syndrome, 32, 41
Multicentric reticulohistiocytosis, 119
Multiple myeloma, 25, 48
Mycobacterium marinum, 131
Mycobacterium leprae, 53, 131
Mycobacterium tuberculosis, 54, 131
Mycosis fungoides, 40, 71, 94, 119
Myocardial infarction, 4

N
Naegeli-Franceschetti-Jadassohn syndrome, 117
Nager syndrome, 117
Nail dystrophy, 9, 99
Naked tubercles, 56
Naproxen, 3
Nasal chondritis, 63
Nasal congestion, 14, 47
Nasal fold papules, 35
Nasal glioma, 37
Nasal obstruction, 38, 53, 56, 71
Nasolacrimal duct stenosis, 136

Neomycin, 92
Neural heterotopia, 37
Neurofibroma, 43, 115, 141
Neurofibromatosis, 43, 119, 148
Neuroma, 30
Neutrophilia, 129
Neutrophilic eccrine hydradenitis, 78
Nevoid basal cell carcinoma syndrome, 31
Nevus flammeus, 7–8, 46, 64, 82, 124, 136, 141
Nevus lipomatosis superficialis, 51
Nevus of Ota, 4–5, 77
Nevus sebaceous, 122–124
New World leishmaniasis, 144
Nicotinic acid, 18
NK (natural killer)/T cell lymphoma, 71
Nodular amyloidosis, 48
Nodular elastoidosis, 48
Nodular scabies, 130
Non-caseating granuloma, 133
Non-Langerhans cell histiocytosis, 32, 44, 119
Noonan syndrome, 51, 136
Norwegian scabies, 100

O
Ochronosis, 3–4, 77
Oculo-auriculo-vertebral spectrum, 137
Oculo-auriculo-vertebral syndrome, 117
Oculocerebrocutaneous syndrome, 118
Odontogenic cyst, 31
Odontogenic keratocyst, 60
Olfactory neuroblastoma, 41
Olmsted syndrome, 99
Omphalocel, 136
Ophtalmic zoster, 12
Ophthalmoplegia, 72
Oral papillomatosis, 65
Orf, 49–50
Organomegaly, 136
Osteochondrodystrophy, 30
Osteoma cutis, 105
Osteomyelitis, 87
Otitis media, 89, 97, 137
Otophyma, 130
Ovarian fibroma, 31

P
Palisaded and encapsulated neuroma, 28
Palmoplantar hyperkeratosis, 23, 65
Palmoplantar keratoderma, 9, 99–100
Palmoplantar pit, 31–32
Palmoplantar punctate keratosis, 107
Panniculitis, 59
Papilloma, 51, 64–65, 107
Papular mucinosis, 34
Paraphenylenediamine, 92
Paraproteinemia, 34
Paroxysmal nocturnal hemoglobinuria, 89
Parvovirus B19, 78
Patch test, 92, 134
Pear-like nose, 66
Pediculosis capitis, 94
Pellagra, 18
Pemphigus foliaceus, 17, 93
Pemphigus seborrheicus, 17
Pemphigus vulgaris, 14, 17, 87
Perichondritis, 80, 115, 131

Perifollicular fibroma, 28
Perioral dermatitis, 6
Periungual fibroma, 29
Perniosis, 105, 108
Petrified ear, 139
PHACES syndrome, 45
Phenytoin, 148
Pheochromocytoma, 30
Phlebectasia, 126
Photoaging, 77
Photoallergic drug reaction, 18
Photodermatosis, 14–15
Photophobia, 7
Photosensitivity, 6–7, 15, 61, 67, 80, 136, 140
Phototoxic drug reaction, 18
Phymatous rosacea, 49, 130
Piebaldism, 5
Pigmented actinic keratosis, 4
Pigmented basal cell carcinoma, 39, 114
Pilomatricoma, 43, 116
Pink disease, 7
Pinocchio nose, 45
Pityriasis alba, 6
Pityriasis rosea, 95
Pityriasis rubra pilaris, 95
Pityriasis versicolor, 77
Plasma cell dyscrasia, 48
Plexiform neurofibroma, 148
Pneumothorax, 29
Poikiloderma, 6–7, 9, 24, 63, 67, 80
Polyarthritis, 80
Polymorphic light eruption, 88, 109
Polyotia, 135
Porokeratosis, 23
Porphyria cutanea tarda, 15, 66, 89, 148
Port-wine stain, 7–8, 46, 82
Posterior fossa malformation, 45
Post-herpetic neuralgia, 12
Postinflammatory hypopigmentation, 6, 77–78
Pox virus, 34, 49
Preauricular pit, 141
Preauricular sinus, 115, 138, 143
Preauricular tag, 118, 138
Pregnancy, 3, 33, 46, 140
Premature aging syndrome, 67, 136
Primary systemic amyloidosis, 48, 105
Progeria, 67, 136
Prolidase deficiency, 63
Pruritus, 7, 11, 14, 19–20, 80, 89, 94, 97,
Pseudolymphoma, 39–40, 119
Pseudomonas aeruginosa, 81
Psoriasis inversa, 95
Psoriasis vulgaris, 20, 94–95
Pulmonary valve stenosis, 136
Purpura fulminans, 144
PUVA therapy, 3
Pyloric atresia, 140
Pyoderma, 13, 86
Pyoderma gangrenosum, 73, 144
Pyogenic granuloma, 46, 125

Q
Quinidine, 3

R
Rabson-Mendenhall syndrome, 65
Radiotherapy, 6, 24, 60, 118, 139, 144

Railroad track ear, 140
Ramsay-Hunt syndrome, 85
Red ear syndrome, 81
Relapsing polychondritis, 63, 80, 140
Renal abnormalities, 115, 118
Renal angiomyolipoma, 30
Renal cell carcinoma, 29, 42
Renal failure, 63
Rendu-Osler-Weber syndrome, 9, 83
Retinoid, 99, 140
Retinoid embryopathia, 140
Rheumatoid arthritis, 134
Rheumatoid nodule, 134
Rhinitis, 35, 55, 62–63, 65, 67, 136
Rhinophyma, 49
Rhinoplasty, 9
Rhinoscleroma, 42, 54, 65
Rhinosporidiosis, 42, 55
Rhinosporidium seeberi, 55
Rodent ulcer, 70
Rosacea, 6, 8, 49, 79, 130
Rosai-Dorfman disease, 33
Rothmund-Thomson syndrome, 6–7, 63, 80, 136–137
Rubinstein-Taybi syndrome, 64
Rudimentary ear, 138

S
Saddle nose, 53, 62–64
Salmon patch, 8
Salt-and-pepper appearance, 136
Sarcoidosis, 35, 56, 63, 133
Sarcoptes scabiei, 100
Scabies, 100, 130
Schwannoma, 46
Scleroatrophy, 9
Sclerodactyly, 9
Scleroderma, 9, 66, 83, 139
Scleromyxedema, 34, 106
Sea blue histiocytosis, 33
Sebaceous adenoma, 32
Sebaceous carcinoma, 41
Sebaceous gland hyperplasia, 30
Seborrheic dermatitis, 18–19, 80, 91–92, 95
Seborrheic keratosis, 4, 35, 50, 102, 122
Segmental lentiginosis, 77
Senile angioma, 33
Senile comedone, 49, 103
Senile sebaceous hyperplasia, 30
Sepsis, 86–87, 138
Septic shock, 73
Septorhinoplasty, 63
Sezary syndrome, 94, 97
Silver sulfadiazine, 4
Sinonasal mucosal melanoma, 38
Sinus tract, 37
Sinusitis, 62, 72
Slapped face, 78
Small ear, 64, 136–137
Small-medium pleomorfic T cell lymphoma, 40
Snap-back elasticity, 137
Solar elastosis, 48, 103
Spastic cerebral palsy, 105
Spicule, 25, 35
Spider angioma, 33
Spindle cell hemangioendothelioma, 46
Spitz nevus, 37–38, 112
Sporotrichosis, 42

Squamous cell carcinoma, 9, 24, 35, 39, 42, 60, 70, 96, 101–102, 120, 139, 143
Staphylococcus aureus, 12
Stevens-Johnson syndrome, 14
Strabismus, 65
Streptococcus pyogenes, 7
Sturge-Weber syndrome, 8
Subependymal nodule, 29
Subepidermal calcified nodule, 105
Sweet's syndrome, 81, 128–129
Swimming pool granuloma, 131
Syndactyly, 64, 118
4p-syndrome, 64
Syphilis, 34, 54, 62, 69, 109
Syringobulbia, 73
Syringoma, 31, 51, 136
Systemic lupus erythematosus (SLE), 6, 21, 79, 81

T
Tabes dorsalis, 73
Tapir nose, 65
Telangiectasia, 7–9, 28, 31, 33, 48–49, 66, 80, 82–83, 116, 124
Thalidomide embryopathia, 140
Thrill, 47, 124
Thromboembolic disease, 109
Thrombocytopenia, 97
Thyroid carcinoma, 29–30
Thyroid dermatopathy, 107
Tinea faciei, 20, 92
Tinnitus, 77, 85
Tin-tack sign, 69
Tophus, 104–105
Topical corticosteroids, 6, 9, 93, 95
Torn earlobes, 135
Townes-Brocks syndrome, 118
Tracheoesophagial fistula, 118
Transverse nasal line, 67
Traumatic hematoma of the auricle, 118
Treacher-Collins syndrome, 115, 118, 138
Treponema pallidum, 54
Treponema pertunea, 62
Trichilemmoma, 30, 107
Trichoblastoma, 123
Trichodiscoma, 28, 107
Trichoepithelioma, 28, 107–108, 116
Trichofolliculoma, 28
Trichorhinophalangeal syndrome, 66
Trichostasis spinulosa, 35
Trigeminal neuritis, 69
Trigeminal trophic syndrome, 73
Trisomy 22 mosaicism, 115
Tryptophan, 18

Tuberculid, 35
Tuberculine test, 54
Tuberculosis, 53–54, 59, 131
Tuberous sclerosis, 29, 49, 108, 115
Turner syndrome, 141
Tzanck cytology, 93

U
Ulerythema ophryogenes, 136
Urticaria, 80
Uveitis, 12

V
VACTERL association, 118
Varicella, 11–12, 85
Varicella zoster virus, 12, 85
Variola-like scar, 15
Vasculitis, 59, 81, 85, 88, 129
Venous lake, 47, 126
Verruca plana, 34–35
Verruca vulgaris, 24
Vertigo, 85
Vitiligo, 5, 78

W
Waardenburg syndrome, 66, 115
Wallenberg syndrome, 73
Warty dyskeratoma, 42
Weathering ear nodules, 104
Wegener's granulomatosis, 62, 88, 133
Werner syndrome, 67
Wilms' tumor, 7
Winer nodule, 105
Wiskott-Aldrich syndrome, 97
Wolf-Hirschhorn syndrome, 64, 118
Wrestler's ear, 118, 140

X
Xanthoma, 105
Xanthoma disseminatum, 32
Xeroderma pigmentosum, 4, 60–61, 77
Xerosis, 63, 65
X-linked dominant chondrodysplasia punctata, 63

Y
Yaws, 62

Z
Zimmermann-Laband syndrome, 141
Zona oticus, 85
Zygomycosis, 72

Printing and Binding: Stürtz GmbH, Würzburg